The Book

Of

A Corporate Yogi

-Ravindra Puri

First Edition: March- 2019

Copyright Material

All rights reserved by the author

Notice

Any information given in this book is not intended to be taken as instructions for yoga, breathing or meditation. Any person intending to learn and practise yoga, breathing techniques or meditation should learn from an expert in the respective area.

Aaditya Books

2018rdp@gmail.com

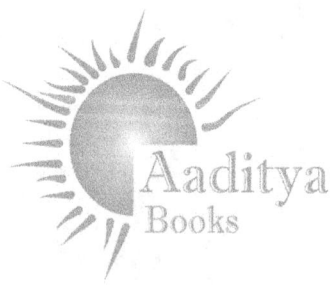

I do not know how I would have finished this book

without the love from my son, Aadi,

without support and motivation from my parents,

learnings from my colleagues and friends in the corporate world

and

direction to a yogic life by yoga gurus.

Praise for The book of a corporate yogi

Today's mundane life revolves around chasing goals, reaching milestones, expanding the network and earning money. The measure of contentment is through achievements, a senior position, and likes on social media. Getting stuck in the vicious circle of fulfilling endless desires, one misses its purpose and being happy at the moment. 'The book of a Corporate Yogi' is an amazing combination of real-life experiences of the author and his evolution. It feels very real as he shares his journey and learnings. It suggests how to be well equipped and be a yogi (centered and peaceful) in chaos. The reassurance- yes, it is possible to be untouched and grow in knowledge while being part of the race. It is a must read.

Ankita Arora,
Art of living teacher, Australia

****

'A Book of Corporate Yogi' is a strong message delivered through references from the ancient Indian practice of Yoga. A simple yet very effective guide on work-life balance. This book is an essential tool for helping readers manage stress, anxiety, and uncertainties through regular practice of Yoga.
While reading 'The book of Corporate Yogi' you might feel it's your own journey narrated by the author; Simple & effective language, choice of words is what makes the book a friend and companion.

Sachin Ganjapurkar,
Supply chain & engineering professional, Singapore

Contents

Foreword

Chapter 1: The need for a yogic life

Chapter 2: Yoga—The journey

Chapter 3: A yogic lifestyle

Chapter 4: Yogic healing

Foreword

At every stage of life, we may feel incomplete. This book will help you to look within yourself to find a sense of completeness or to reduce the sense of incompleteness. The human mind is like a jar, and just like a half-filled jar makes noise because of its part-emptiness, similarly our minds make noise because of the feeling of incompleteness. The noise made by the mind is the reason for all the chaos we can feel in life.

The life of a corporate employee is always difficult and it always has been. Ambitious goals can add to the feeling of incompleteness. In our lives, most of us encounter struggles, hardships, frustration, pain, heartache, anxiety, loneliness and broken relationships. While we often think that we are the only one facing these problems, everyone is fighting their own battle. It is not the problem of modern life. It has been there since inception. The only difference is that in modern life we have started ignoring how to handle it.

Corporate employees live their lives in a rat race, and suddenly one day they find themselves in a crisis. It could be an illness, stress, financial problems or whatever. That's when people start exploring alternate ways to handle their situation. But not everyone will be lucky enough to find the solution. Learning a yogic way of living and making minor modifications in lifestyle can bring happiness, peace of mind and clarity of thoughts. There is more need to be a yogi in the corporate world now than ever before because of the stress, pressure and pace of life expected of us.

In the corporate world you will find many people who are conscious (or at least try or pretend to be) about what they eat. People find time to go for a walk or fit in a quick bout of exercise, which is a really good thing, but their mental health is completely neglected. Few make the effort to understand their own mental health. Mental health is often confused with your mood. Some think that listening to songs, partying, drinking alcohol or smoking cigarettes are quick remedies to maintain their mental health. But that is like taking aspirin when you have headache. You may feel immediate relief but the issues can surface again because the root cause hasn't been dealt with.

We live in a corporate world where nothing is permanent. Some say there is nothing called a permanent job anymore. The moment we lose a job, we are empty-handed. Our hands remain empty because when we have a title and salary, we just focus on the power of that title and earn money. What we forget is to earn people, happiness and health. We forget to earn happiness as we confuse ourselves with the definition of happiness and get stuck on the merry-go-round of pain and pleasure. What we think will bring pleasure (such as material things) will ultimately land us in pain. Glorified business models, theories and philosophies do not address this problem.

The corporate world has become like a factory, where no one knows you before you join and after your exit. Alexander the Great had a similar ambition to the corporates—conquer the world even though you don't know where the world ends. And one day, during the journey, just like Alexander, something or someone will remind us of the stark reality of life, in that while chasing ambition you left behind your happiness. You became unhappy in search of happiness. Whatever struggle you go through will only land in unhappiness, and one day things will suddenly end, leaving a feeling of regret for an unlived life. There is no return path to go back on to correct the mistakes you've made in your life. But it's never too late. Unfortunately, no one teaches that happiness is not in the future—it is in the present moment. People ask whether you have a job, family, house, car, money, but no one asks whether you are happy.

Becoming a yogi can help you to understand the meaning and purpose of life. It allows you to discover the wholeness of life. How not to be impacted by the ups and downs of life and how to achieve inner peace. It allows you to find a new world. Becoming a yogi does not mean to wear saffron clothes and renounce everything. You can be a corporate yogi. Corporate yoginess is about being happy while being in the chaotic corporate world, and taking good care of your own self.

Many management philosophies speak the same language as yogic practices. I have drawn a parallel with management philosophies and models throughout the book. In some cases, yogic practices bring more insights into why these management models should be followed, and in other cases yogic practices add more value to the existing models. Yogic practices can bring a huge difference to many areas of corporate life. They also fill the gaps not addressed by management models and concepts.

Humans created alphabets from A to Z, and drew boundaries on the Earth. Now our whole world and emotions revolve around these letters and the sentences created using them. Our world is defined by boundaries drawn by us. There is a world before the A to Z and beyond the boundaries created by us. A to Z, or the world with boundaries, is just the subgroup created for our convenience. This book talks about going beyond the commonly known world.

Well-known yogi Jaggi Vasudev once mentioned that approximately two billion people around the world practise yoga, fundamentally, "because it works". So, we don't have to reinvent the wheel to find the path to happiness. Yogic life is a proven path to happiness.

"The Book of a Corporate Yogi" tries to address the gaps of existing business models and corporate philosophies and highlights the yogic practices that can make life easier.

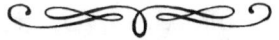

Chapter 1

The need for a yogic life

In 2008, almost the whole world was grappling with the great recession. The fall of Lehman Brothers sent a panic throughout the world. While watching the news and its effects on many lives in the United States and other developed countries, I hadn't realised that it had reached my doorstep too. Suddenly, the mood of the people who shared the bus to my office started changing. There were noticeable silences and forced smiles on their faces. People started murmuring and justifying why they wouldn't be affected. And then there was the first casualty. One of my friends was "asked to go home". That's the term that was used instead of redundancy. The reasons given were ambiguous; mainly related to performance, partly related to slow business, etc. But we all knew. It was the recession. It was spreading like a plague. The next day, there was one more casualty, and it continued. Seeing someone on the bus meant they had survived that day; that's how life became. There was no question of finding a job outside the current organisation as the whole industry was struggling. Expats were returning to their home countries. The feeling was as if the air was filled with gloom. People losing their jobs in the corporate had a massive effect on all the industries. The whole market, as well as life, seemed to be slowing down.

One of my mentors was a senior experienced professional. I caught up with him for a coffee to seek his guidance about how I should approach this situation. When we met, to my great surprise, he had teary eyes. He had recently bought a home with a mortgage. And he had just been told by his organisation that he was no longer needed. His kids had just entered university. Mortgage, kids' education... There was a huge financial burden on him, and suddenly he had been asked to leave the organisation. After we'd talked, I wished him well and left with a heavy heart, but I also felt lucky—I had bought a property with a mortgage that wasn't a huge burden at the time as my parents were supportive, and I had no other financial burdens on me. Even if I had lost my job, I would have survived for a few months. But then a thought struck me: how long can I be lucky? Not always... My parents wouldn't always be there to support me. I saw many people whose careers were termed a success, tumbling down to the ground. How was I going to make sure that I would never face that situation in my life?

I looked at the economic cycles and realised that recession is not a one-time event. It's a cyclic event. It's always going to pop up every now and then. I became quieter as I lost my direction. My professors who had taught me how to succeed in corporate life were silent too.

A normal thing happened: I started smoking more cigarettes. I say normal because that's what we do in the corporate world to get rid of our stress. I started drinking more, too, to avoid the thoughts of an uncertain future. One day, one of my friends asked me to try yoga. I had no inclination towards a spiritual life, and I mentioned that to my friend. He tried explaining that yoga is not about becoming spiritual but is about taking care of your own health. I wasn't convinced and had no intention of falling prey to some marketing gimmick. But then he played his final stroke: he asked me to join a yoga class, and if I didn't see the benefits, then he would pay for it. And then he played an emotional card, too, saying he was my friend and that he would never suggest any wrong thing to me. I had to surrender. I enrolled for a program called the "Happiness Program". The title itself brought a smile to my face. It was a five-day program and it was in the evening after my office hours, so I wouldn't have any difficulty attending it.

Day one, Monday, just before I entered the program room, I smoked, just to get some extra energy or something to get me through sitting in that program. Yes, I was probably nervous. After day one, I was hooked on the concept of achieving happiness through yogic ways. I was a regular smoker but didn't even get the urge to smoke for the next two days. A smoker taking a break from smoking for a few days or sometimes even for a few months is not uncommon. On the Wednesday after the class, I had the urge for a smoke. I bought the cigarette out of the packet and lit it. I smoked half the cigarette and suddenly felt

14

as though I was forcing myself to smoke it. And I stopped. That was the last time in my life I smoked. I never again had the urge to smoke after that. I felt happy. I felt no need to depend on external substances to reduce my stress. Over a period of time, I realised that not only my body had started developing a resistance to smoking, and then alcohol, but my mind had also started developing a resistance to stress arising from small and petty things.

There is a need of yogic life to answer all those unanswered questions in our mind.

We have been living in the modern world full of technology that we feel has made our lives easier. Still, the pain we feel, the joy, sadness and other emotions haven't changed. Merely the physical things around us have changed. When we move from an office that uses less technology to an office that uses a lot of technology, it can seem to make us feel happy for some time, but that feeling is momentary. We still struggle to find the answers to questions like, Who am I? Where am I going? What's happening to my life? And we turn to an internet search engine as the one to give us the answers to all our questions. In reality, all answers are within our body and mind—we just need to ask them. When we don't get the answers to our questions, we feel lost. Feeling lost arises when we don't know where we are going. It's like you are in the middle of a desert and your GPS stops functioning, and you feel lost. That's exactly what happens when we don't know where we are going in our personal life. It's like the difference between speed and velocity. You may have speed, not the velocity. (Velocity is speed with direction.) You don't know where the speed will take you; hence, the need for velocity.

I was invited to do an alumnus talk in the university where I had completed my graduation. I was told to choose my favourite topic for my talk. That's when I started thinking: what is my favourite topic? When I was in university, I was known for my love of trees, event management and innovation. By this stage, however, I hadn't planted a tree in years, I hadn't organised any events, nor worked on any innovations. That's when I started struggling to understand my favourite subject. Was wearing a suit and carrying a fancy title my favourite thing? Not really because many times I had tried to stay away from it. The question made my mind blank, and I started thinking: Who am I? What am I doing? What are my goals? Someone asked me what my favourite flower was. I took quite some time to even come up with an answer. But even though after thinking for a while I told them about my favourite flower, I was not sure whether it really was my favourite flower. Many times, we have favourites just to show them to the rest of the world, but reality can be different. You may name an expensive perfume as your favourite fragrance, just to make sure you create a certain impression on the people around you, but the reality could be that you just like the fragrance of a sea breeze or the fragrance of soil after the first rain of the wet season.

When you ask questions like "Who am I?", it means you haven't spent enough time with yourself to understand yourself. What we say our favourites are to the rest of the world could be different than what we really believe them to be.

What is your favourite colour, flower, location, author, movie, hobby, etc.? Spend some time thinking about this. The moment you get the answers will tell you more about you to yourself. You will realise that these things bring happiness to you. If it doesn't bring happiness, it's not your favourite. The Johari window concept addresses this dilemma well. The Johari window technique was developed by psychologist Joseph Luft and Harrington Ingham in 1955. It helps to understand the relationship of people with themselves and with others. The technique is widely used in relationship management in the work environment.

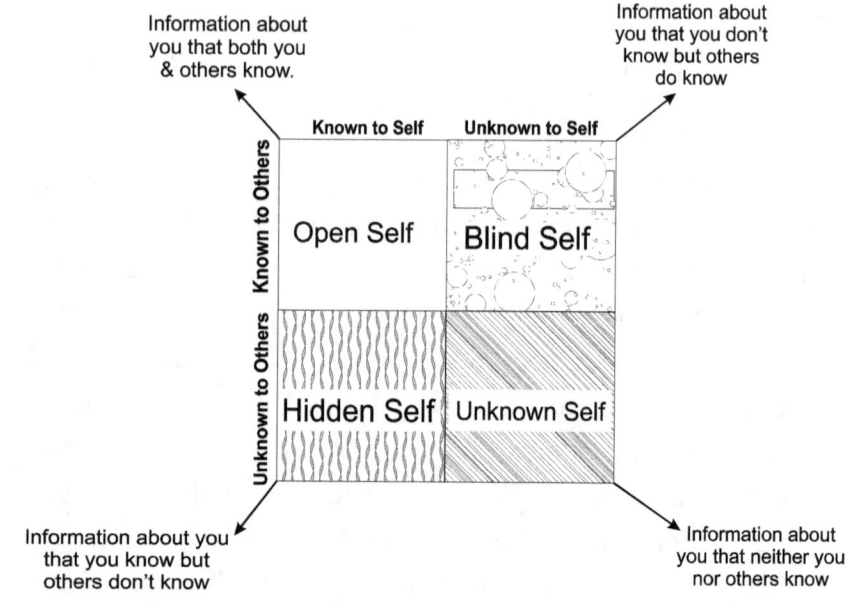

Fig. Johari Window

The focus is on:

1. Open self: correcting your open self if it has some obvious shortcomings, such as aggressive behaviour.
2. Blind self: making you aware of your blind self; for example, some habits that you may not think are bad but could be bad.
3. Hidden self: making some of your good characteristics known to others. For example, you might be a good writer but you have never shown this skill to the rest of the world.

4. Unknown self: this is an aspect about yourself that you never knew, and others don't know about it either. For example, you come across something accidentally and realise that that's what makes you happy.

Current management programs and self-help initiatives do not focus much on exploring the unknown self. The unknown self is also known as a black hole because you don't know what's inside it. It's like a coal mine with huge reserves of precious metals. It takes pain, effort and time to find it but, once found, it has a hugely positive impact on our lives.

Yogic life helps to explore the region "Not known to others, not known to self"—the unknown self.

The trap

A simple question to ask yourself is:

"When will I be happy?"

If you ask this question to someone in a workplace, you will most probably receive answers like:

"When I become a manager."

"When I earn X amount of salary."

Keep repeating the question and you will realise that there are a few more things that need to be achieved to be happy. Answers could include:

"When I am in perfect health."

"When I have no liabilities."

"When my kids go to university."

And you will realise that the list will never be finished. Interestingly, many people achieve many things that they feel will make them happy, but find the happiness is only momentary.

Answers to the question also vary depending on various factors, such as age, gender and geography.

Will you be happy if you become the CEO of the organisation?

If your answer is yes then all CEOs would be the happiest people on Earth.

Will you be happy if you earn a lot of money?

If yes, then all the richest people would be the happiest.

So, if the topmost position in the organisation cannot guarantee happiness, and if money cannot assure you joy, then what exactly are we trying to achieve?

It's a trap.

A corporate person tends to get stuck in two types of traps:

1.   Happiness trap

2. Social trap

Happiness trap:

Me and some friends were camping at a free campsite in northern Queensland, Australia, one November. There was a campfire that lots of people gathered around at night-time. Some sang, or played musical instruments, some danced, some just enjoyed the fire and the surroundings, and some chatted. We met a German girl who was backpacking around Australia. When she realised we were travelling to Airlie Beach she asked if we had space for one more in our car as she wanted to go there too, but her other travel mates wanted to spend time in a different area. Luckily, we had some space so we offered her a lift. Her name was Liz (short for Elizabeth) and she had just recently graduated. She was from a poor family and never thought that she would be able to visit Australia. Her father's health was not too good so she was finding it difficult to stay away from her family. Somehow, she managed.

She was travelling on a shoestring budget; living in hostels, and sometimes working in hostels in lieu of accommodation. She had managed to keep aside money if she needed to go back to Germany in case of an emergency. The best part of her travel was that she was enjoying every part of it. Even if she had to work as a cleaning assistant, she still enjoyed that work because the money took care of her travel costs. At times, she worked on farms to get more money. But whatever she was doing she was enjoying it. She had just one year and she wanted to see the whole of Australia in that year. She wasn't sure whether she would ever be able to come back. She didn't have time to complain about anything; she just wanted to travel at any cost and live her dream. I liked how she ignored the hardships and looked at living life for that one year. After finishing that year, she had travelled the whole of Australia and went back to Germany with lots of memories and a lifetime of experience before embarking on her postgraduate studies.

Even after finishing her travels she continued a similar perspective towards her life. She was of the opinion that she had a limited time to live (although she was healthy and young), and she wanted to live her life to its fullest without getting bothered about the hardships and setbacks.

Many people miss the happiness that people like Liz find. In the corporate world we often live the exact opposite life to Liz. When we are at work, we are part of work and forget ourselves. We also tend to forget that there is life outside work as we spend the maximum time at work. And the only things we chase are small pleasures, like a promotion or salary increments. We consider that these things will bring happiness, yet these pleasures hardly last a few days. Office politics, dominating each other, power struggles; they all become the means to achieve happiness, which never happens. That's why it is a trap; a happiness trap.

Social trap:

There is a word in Japanese, "Johatsu", which means evaporated people. It's not physical evaporation, but is the term used for those thousands of Japanese people tormented by the shame of a lost job, failed marriage or mounting debt, who have reportedly started leaving behind their formal identities and seeking refuge in the anonymous, off-the-map world. This is a parallel society in Japan where you can live life without letting others know about it by changing your name, address, work, etc. Basically, it's starting a new life with a clean slate. In a way it takes away the social pressures and the people can live the life they want.

There was a famous incident that showed how people disappeared overnight from society. A man from Tokyo had been fired from his accounting job but was too ashamed to tell his family and friends. Each morning he would put on his shirt and tie, kiss his wife and kid goodbye and travel in the direction of his office. But without a place to go to he instead spent all day in a garden, sometimes staying late to give the impression there was extra work on or that he was drinking with his colleagues. This continued for a couple of months. Finally, as there was no salary coming in, he could not continue the lie. One day he left his house, never to return, and just vanished, disappearing in Sanya, which is a place known as a parallel society to those who want to wipe out their identity from society.

It is easy to do this in Japan because Japanese law maintains the privacy of information of people's whereabouts, except in criminal offences. The trend was more apparent during the 1990 financial crisis.

Because Japan has a name for this situation, it has become popular, but in fact it exists in every part of the world. The first symptom of Johatsu is burnout because of work pressures and office politics. The easiest escape people find is to change their job. The next level would be changing their career, changing the country, and so on. So, when people can't change their identity they try to change their surroundings, where they find it difficult to survive with their own identity. Johatsu is present everywhere but in different forms. The Western world has many such social groups that live untraditional lives. America has seen the hippy era. Various cults are also examples of Johatsu, where people want to live life away from society's norms.

The question is, why can't we all live the life we want? Because it's a social trap. Any event that is different from what society expects can bring shame, and that's how we get into the social trap. We finish our education, start earning money, get married, have children and die. This looks like a normal cycle. Whereas if you don't go to school and pursue a career, if you don't earn enough money, if you don't get married or if you get divorced, if you lose your job, etc.; all this is considered shameful.

The reality is that you will never be able to meet society's expectations because they are superficial:

- If you don't have money, they will call you poor.
- If you have lots of money, they will call you arrogant rich.
- You are illiterate if you don't study.
- You are a bookworm if you study a lot.
- Working hard in an office makes you someone with no interest in a personal life.
- Taking work easily makes you less ambitious.
- You are thought to be stupid if you don't come up with ideas.
- You are thought to be over-smart if you come up with lots of ideas.
- People will blame you anyway.

So live your life!

There was an old farmer who lived in a village. One year there was less rainfall than normal and not enough for the crop to survive the year. The farmer decided to sell one of his horses to get some money to support his family.

That day, he left for the market with his ten-year-old son. They both rode on the horse. People on the way looked at them and pitied the horse, saying how ruthless the father and son were, both riding on a poor horse. So the farmer decided to let his son alone ride the horse. Another group of people saw them and said how sad it was that the old father had to walk while the child rode the horse, and they pitied the farmer. The farmer decided to ride the horse and let his son walk. A few onlookers mentioned how shameful it was that the child was walking while the father was comfortably enjoying the ride. This time the farmer decided to walk along with his son and the horse. People started laughing at him because he had a horse but wasn't using it. So, finally, the farmer decided to carry the horse. He tied its legs to a strong stick and father and son started carrying the horse. They were crossing a bridge on a river when the horse started panicking. It thought they were going to kill him, so it frantically tried to free itself and struggled. All three lost their balance and fell into the river and died.

No matter what you do, people will find faults in your actions. Don't fall for the social trap!

Choosing the right course at the right time

It was the end of a long day at work. Exhausted, I packed my bags and left. I entered the elevator and met this gentleman who happened to be a new employee in the organisation. After exchanging greetings and small-talk, he offered me a lift in his car as we both lived in the same suburb. I was happy to accept. He told me that he was an ex-Air Force pilot. He was probably the first Air Force pilot I had met in my life, and I told him so. I was curious to know why he left the Air Force and joined the corporate world. His smiled conveyed that he was comfortable answering my question. He told me that flying was his passion, but something had happened and so he had taken a break from it. Now I was even more curious to know the story of why he'd left flying.

As an Air Force pilot, he had to do routine practices. One day, a fleet of fighter jets flew a routine practice, covering a predefined route. This gentleman was flying one of the modern high-speed jets. A couple of minutes into the flight he had some technical issues. He was alone on the flight. He started receiving instructions from air traffic control (ATC) and he started following those instructions. All of a sudden, something unexpected happened. The glass canopy above his head opened and he started feeling the huge wind pressure on his face and the rest of his body. It was like someone was pressing his head against a glass wall. He felt numb and motionless. He couldn't hear anything from ATC. He was in that situation for only a couple of seconds when he felt that his life was over. Pictures of his family flew in front of his eyes and he became teary. He collected himself and tried to focus on the instructions from ATC. Somehow, he managed to follow the instructions, and landed safely. There was no explosion, and not even a single scratch on his body. The moment he landed he was surrounded by emergency response vehicles. He was immediately pulled out of the jet and taken to hospital. He could not utter a single word for the next hour or so. He was in shock. After some time, he realised that one of his close friends was waving at him, and tears started rolling from his eyes. He realised that he was alive; those were tears of happiness.

When I was listening to this story, I felt as if my whole body was freezing. I experienced and lived those moments with him. This gentleman told me that the incident taught him an important lesson in life. He said life is like a flight. You know the starting point and the end point. What is not sure is the path in between. And it is not a straight path between the starting point and the end point of life either. The success of life, and success of flight, depends on how you respond to the various situations, and how you change the course of your life or flight at the right time to avoid a crash.

The key to success in life is choosing the right course at the right time, and many times we feel the need for assistance.

A Harvard lesson that I learned in Hervey Bay

There was a time in my life when I had quit my job and literally had no plans for my future.

After sitting quietly for a week or so, I decided to go on a road trip in my car with a minimum budget. I had no money for hotels and restaurants, which meant I had to do free camping, low-cost hostels and cook my own food.

I travelled all the way from Sydney to Hervey Bay. Hervey Bay is known for its proximity to Fraser Island; the world's biggest sand island. After reaching Hervey Bay, I immediately went to Fraser

Island and spent three days on that beautiful and unique island. It was a lifetime experience in itself. Then I returned to Hervey Bay.

After taking a nice afternoon nap, my body was craving a hot cup of coffee. I made a cup of coffee for myself and sat in a hammock in the open space of the hostel.

There were two women a little way away from me. One of them was scribbling something in her diary while the other was browsing through a book. Probably a Lonely Planet.

I finished my coffee and joined them. Travel makes you more extroverted. I had already started experiencing these changes in me. My "Hello" turned into an in-depth conversation. These women were Harvard graduates. For a business management graduate like myself, this was a pleasant surprise. This was also my first interaction with someone from Harvard Business School. At the same time, I found it hard to digest the fact that Harvard graduates were staying in a hostel.

"Personal transformation", perhaps one of the women read my mind as she said, "We're on a personal transformation journey."

Personal transformation—this sounded like Harvard-type jargon to me.

"Have you ever wondered, 'Who am I? What am I doing? Where am I going?' If the answer is yes then personal transformation is the key," she said.

Suddenly, I felt like lots of bells were ringing in my head. I had been trying to find answers to these questions for so long and now this woman was giving me the answers to my own questions without me even asking them out loud.

Every individual gets into a habit of routine. Every day you get up in the morning, go to work, do work, attend meetings, come home, and call it a day. And the cycle continues. The result is lots of stress, anxiety and sometimes depression. Look at how many people suffer from stress, anxiety or these kinds of issues and you will understand exactly what I am saying.

Personal transformation is the answer.

How do you feel when you read a book or visit a new place or learn a new skill? You feel good, right? Why is that? Because it releases the feel-good hormone—endorphins.

Breaking the routine pattern is the key.

When you play with a kid, you act like a kid, you jump like a kid, and you laugh like a kid. Why is that? For that short duration you transform yourself into a kid. When you learn a new skill you become an artist. When you plan an outdoor game, you become a sportsperson. You may not be good at sports, but when you are playing that sport you behave like a sportsperson. You may be an executive in your organisation but when you play the game you become a sportsperson. That's personal transformation—transforming yourself completely from your current situation.

Breaking the routine pattern *regularly* is the key.

When I quit my job, I did not have a word for my action. Inadvertently, I was seeking a personal transformation. Until then I had still felt some guilt about quitting my well-paid job, but after that discussion, it just disappeared. This is the lesson on personal transformation that a Harvard graduate taught me in Hervey Bay.

The corporate world contributes to emotions like fear, anxiety, weakness, doubt, hatred, insecurity and stress. Personal transformation is about turning all these emotions into exactly the opposite.

The real crisis

I once visited Bali, Indonesia. The city of Ubud has an amazing market and I was enjoying the shopping. I entered a bag shop and enquired about a man-bag. I wanted to buy a particular type of man-bag. The shop did not have what I wanted but still, out of curiosity, I continued looking at their variety of bags. The shop owner was a sweet Balinese lady. With a pleasant smile, she asked me, "Where did you come from?" Without delay I answered, "Australia". With a naughty expression, she replied, in a Balinese tone, "Nooooo, you are Indian!" I was a bit surprised with this reaction and it brought a smile to my face. But I felt an identity crisis. I had just answered what she had asked. But for a moment I was like, "Who am I?" Indian or Australian... Anyway, I told her that, yes, I am Indian but now I live in Australia. So I come from Australia. That made her happy.

When an actor performs in a movie, he/she takes on another identity. But at the end of the day, they come back to their real identity. In the corporate world we take on different roles, which give us identities different to the real us. Someone could be really humble but will act the opposite in a work environment because of their role. The further we go from the real us, the more we feel lost and the more we get the urge to return back to the real us. Therefore, in the corporate world, we live in a sort of compromised reality. The real trouble starts when we have to act against our real nature, perhaps because of the title we have in the corporate world, which creates this sense of duality. All life's sufferings can be said to be the result of the mental chaos that arises from the sense of duality. When we are experiencing the conflict from duality, our entire life becomes painful, and we do not know a moment's peace. It becomes a case of cognitive dissonance.

The phenomenon of cognitive dissonance is about holding two conflicting ideas or behaviours simultaneously in a conscious mind. Often, the uncomfortable disagreement that results from the situation is joined by an internal drive towards justification of the idea or behaviour by rationalising it. Thus, smokers know that smoking is not good for their health, but keep smoking by justifying that smoking keeps their weight lower. In a similar way, we often come to understand the proper healthy lifestyle that can result from living a yogic life, but are still willing to risk cognitive dissonance by constantly falling off the good health wagon in our quest for perceived happiness. That is the duality of the mind.

The following factors may contribute to the duality of the mind:

1. Knowledge
2. Misconception
3. Past experiences
4. Memory
5. Sleep

These factors need to be studied so as to understand and control the duality of the mind. You may argue, what is the need to discuss or consider sleep, memory, etc.? Sleep is sleep or memory is memory. However, poor memory can impact decisions and a good memory can bring joy. Lack of sleep might affect the other four areas. If you don't get enough sleep, it can impact your memory, it can create misconceptions. So it is important to understand these factors and their impact on life. Interestingly, all these factors have a close relationship with our mind.

Yogic practices divide sleep into three types:

1. Tamasic: you feel heavy, lethargic and dull after sleep.

2. Rajasic: disturbed, irritated, restless sleep.
3. Satvic: sleep that brings lightness, brightness and freshness.

The ultimate goal of yogic practice is to have Satvic sleep.

We return to innocence in sleep. No sleeper can be a sinner. The goal of a student of yoga is to transform this into a positive state of mind while we are awake.

What is the reality?

Six Sigma is a highly structured and effective problem-solving methodology. Many organisations, such as General Electric and Motorola, boast financial success as a result of organisation-wide use of this methodology. Six Sigma uses statistics to decide the solutions to problems. When I was studying my Six Sigma Black Belt course, my professor was really amazing and tried explaining all the fundamentals of complex statistical tools. Nowadays, we have advanced software that makes our lives easier and we don't have to do the tedious calculations manually.

One day we were taught how to create a regression model. This is one of the statistical models normally used for forecasting. It is a fairly complex tool to build manually. After spending several hours learning how to build a regression model, my professor was happy with the outcome, and then he commented, "Lies, damn lies and statistics!"

We had spent hours building that complex model and the professor said there was still a probability that it may not be correct. For the first time in my life I realised that no matter how much you know, there is still something beyond what you know, and that is the real mystery of life because we don't know how much we don't know!

Even with modern medical science there are no solutions to many illnesses. If someone suffers from something, they go to their doctor. The doctor does some tests and may ask you to see a specialist. There are thousands of diseases where a specialist could diagnose or confirm something that would be irreversible. All medicines are given based on probability, and there is still a chance that we might not be lucky. That's the mystery.

We live between the sky and the earth. We look at the sky and we think we know about the sky; the stars, clouds, colour, sun, moon, etc. That's it. We have an understanding of some of the stars and galaxy. And then we reach out at speculation at what could be there beyond the galaxies.

We stand on the earth. We know about earth, soil, the different layers, to a certain extent. We don't know beyond that.

Quantum physics is a fundamental theory that describes nature at the smallest scale of energy levels of atoms and subatomic particles. What does quantum physics tell us about the world? According to the Copenhagen interpretation, this question has a simple answer: quantum physics tells us nothing whatsoever about the world.

There is a knowable world that we understand through study and experience, but probably what we know is still tiny compared to the unknowable world.

If we agree with this principle, the same thing applies in our corporate life. We see lots of decisions being taken in the organisation and we spend hours speculating the reasons behind those decisions with the knowable world. What we keep forgetting, before jumping to conclusions, is that we don't know what we don't know.

We can close our eyes and take a tour of a place to experience it, and other times we can physically be at the place but still not notice the beauty of it. So the question arises: does the world exist outside our head or inside our head? Many times, the worst situations that our minds think will never happen in our life, and things that we never think could happen, suddenly one day do. Medical science has dissected the brain, but couldn't find anything called a mind. Our mind is probably the most mysterious thing in the world.

Mind affects body

In the movie *Shrek*, when Shrek and Donkey are crossing the bridge to go to the castle to free Princess Fiona, Donkey is okay if he doesn't look down through the bridge. But when he looks down, his legs start trembling. The situation did not change, but his mind created that impact on his body.

The way people train in a circus to kill fear in the mind is really interesting. Initially, they put a plank on the ground and ask the participant to walk over it. Then they blindfold the participant and raise the plank into the air and ask the participant to walk over it again. The participant is comfortable walking over the plank in both situations. Then they take the blindfold off and ask the participant to walk on the elevated plank. This time the participant will tremble. The situation did not change but the mind impacted the performance.

The mind, has a habit of going to the extreme (fight or flight), which impacts our decisions. The key is to keep the mind stable. Most of the worst fears imagined will never happen.

The beautiful and the ugly

"Your top is really nice, where did you buy it from?" This is a common comment heard and said many times over. Many times, it is just a conversation starter with someone, which actually has nothing to do with the thing they're praising. Should these comments really bother you?

You don't see yourself unless you stand in front of a mirror. We don't watch ourselves sleeping in bed, curled up silent with our chests rising and falling with our own rhythm. We don't see ourselves reading a book, watching a drama with our eyes fluttering and glowing. We don't see ourselves looking at someone with love and care in our hearts. There is no mirror in our way when we are laughing and smiling and pure happiness is leaking out of us. You would know how bright and beautiful you are if you saw yourself in the moments where you are your truly authentic self.

The question is: who decides whether you are beautiful or ugly? And should someone else's opinion bother you?

In the corporate environment, no doubt you've come across a "performance improvement plan" (PIP), which is a tool to give an employee with perceived performance deficiencies. Many times, this term is misused to pressurise team members to consider resigning. This kind of situation is common especially when a manager doesn't like a team member. In reality, the manager could be incompetent or the team member has more knowledge. In that case, the performance improvement plan is just a device and it doesn't actually mean your performance is poor. Just because the manager thinks that the team member is poor, doesn't make him or her poor.

The key is to not let others' opinions bother you. Life is easier when we understand that a praising comment or an insulting comment may or may not be real. It's like avoiding being a football of others' opinions.

We create the external world

If we say that we create the external world, it may sound difficult to digest. We don't create the trees, sun and moon, but, at the same time, we do decide what is good and what is bad, what is a day and what is a night, what is the sun and what is the moon, what is ugly and what is beautiful.

A teenager who thinks drinking alcohol is a good thing may have parents who think drinking alcohol is a bad thing. Someone may think eating dog is acceptable, someone else may think eating dog is the cruellest thing in the world. Someone thinks that there is a god; someone else thinks there is nothing called God. Someone sees beauty in the ocean; someone else is scared of the ocean.

What is good for one person, could be bad for another.

We name this choice as a culture. Our culture is our world and we create it by fitting things around us into it in the way we want. That's how we create our own world.

"Peace and happiness cannot come from the external world, but comes from within."

Many cultures have traditions. These help its members look inward to find happiness. Sometimes this is in the form of religious rituals or festivals. Unfortunately, many good practices have been distorted over time and have lost their original intent. On the other hand, many practices have been dubbed superstitions without their importance and the science behind them being understood.

In many countries there is a tradition of offering water to guests when they come into your home. In many religions it is required that you clean your feet before worshipping God. The logical mind challenges why you need to clean only your feet when your whole body could be sweaty. Does this challenge make sense? What we forget is that the skin of the human body is also an organ. It helps us to understand touch. It protects our internal body from the external environment. When we put our body to extra work, it takes away pressure from the kidneys by secreting sweat. The skin on our feet does this function perfectly. If we don't clean our feet regularly, we prevent the proper functioning of the skin. So when we come from the outside, and clean the feet, we make sure that our feet remain in the best position to keep functioning. When we pour cold water on our feet, it also relaxes the nervous system and helps us to calm down.

It is important to identify right practices and make use of the external world to find peace within.

Midcareer crisis

The term "midcareer crisis" is becoming more popular day by day. People start their careers as fresh graduates, often with a short-term goal to earn more money and higher designations within organisations. Your late twenties and early thirties are spent slogging for these goals, often forgetting everything else.

When you start earning good money and reach a senior level, that's when you start feeling that you have hit the glass ceiling. You can still try harder to earn more money and higher designations, but soon you start realising that it doesn't make a difference in your life. That's when you realise that you are in a midcareer crisis.

You no longer feel excited about your current role. You get stuck with the dilemma—what do I do next? You start exploring other career options. I have seen many training modules talk about how to choose a new career path. But none of them talk about how you will become happy after choosing a new career path. The biggest question remains unanswered: what is the guarantee that the new career path will give the happiness you are looking for? That's where the talk about risk appetite and taking a risk in life comes in. You take the risk of leaving the already-built career behind, and if you struggle to succeed you still work really hard because you don't want to be seen as a failure in the eyes of society. That's when you spend the rest of your life with an external layer of happiness. Some might go back to their old career, a handful will do great in their new career. It's a risk indeed.

It's not that taking risk is bad, or that changing your career is bad. But making decisions without understanding the root cause behind them can be bad. If your aim is to be happy, then changing your career can contribute to this, but it is not always the solution.

Does only experience bring knowledge?

My friends and I were exploring the northern Queensland region of Australia, and when we reached Bundaberg, we didn't know much about the area except for the Bundaberg rum factory. The weather wasn't good; it was raining heavily. In heavy rains, we visited the factory and saw the amazing process of making rum. We were told about the famous beach called Mon Repos (my rest) where loggerhead sea turtles come and lay eggs. We decided to visit that beach.

We reached the beach in the evening. As it was not a pre-planned visit, we bought the entry tickets after arriving. The beach was managed by volunteers. There were people who had booked tickets a couple of days before. They put visitors into groups to avoid crowding on the beach and to not bother the turtles. As we'd only got tickets on arrival, we were placed in the last of three groups. The most probable time for the turtles to visit the beach was after 11 pm. We mentally prepared ourselves for a long wait as it was only 7 pm when we arrived. Meanwhile, the volunteers played documentaries about the life of sea turtles and we realised what a great job these people were doing in preserving the turtles from vanishing.

When turtles are born they leave the beach on their own and travel thousands of kilometres away from their birthplace. Female sea turtles reach puberty at the age of twenty. When it's time for laying eggs they come to the same beach where they were born. That is an incredible phenomenon. They could be hundreds of kilometres away from their birth beach but they come back to the same beach to lay their eggs. It's like they have natural GPS in their body, which guides them back to the same location.

It was 11.30 pm and still no sign of any sea turtles. Volunteers patrolled the beach throughout the night to keep track of the turtles. At 12.30 am, all three groups were called onto the beach just to avoid disappointment and restlessness. We were close to twenty visitors. One of the volunteers engaged us in conversation, giving more information about the place. Then his walky-talky beeped with the message that a sea turtle had been sighted coming up the beach. We were all instructed not to make any noise, not to use phones and to avoid any light, and not to bother the turtles in their natural process. Understanding the egg-hatching process, none of us wanted to do anything to disturb the turtles.

We reached the turtle as it was moving up the beach away from the water to find a suitable spot. We were thrilled to see it in its natural habitat. Its pace was slow as she was cumbersome out of the water as well as carrying the weight of her eggs. I'm sure it was difficult for her, but she was adamant to find a safe place for her babies. Finally, she found a place and, with her legs, she started digging up the sand. She dug a hole of more than a foot deep. When she was satisfied with the depth, she started laying the eggs, one after another, probably up to a hundred. Once she was done, she carefully buried the eggs with the sand. She looked back at the place where her eggs were buried before she started moving back towards the water. I was moved when I thought she would never see her babies. Before getting into the water, she looked back once again, before slowly getting into the surf and letting the tides pull her out into the ocean.

The volunteers made sure that the eggs were covered properly with the sand to protect them from dogs, vultures, etc. I really admired their work. Once the eggs hatched, the little turtles would dig up to the surface, then start crawling to the ocean. They would keep crawling and the lucky ones who were not spotted by predators would swim away into the ocean.

And the cycle continues.

What a beautiful experience. We kept wondering about the whole process. No one taught the turtles what to do.

Experience is not the only thing that gives us knowledge; we have inherent knowledge in ourselves. One of which is creativity. The question is: what do we do to explore it? The other question is: do we also do something to suppress it?

What is your raison d'être?

It's a myth that you should have one goal; you need to have at least 100 goals in life. What is your goal in life? This question is often a struggle to answer.

If your ultimate goal is to get a good job, what happens when you get the good job? The definition of "good" keeps changing.

If your goal is to earn good money, what happens when you earn good money? The definition of earning good money keeps changing.

That's what happens when you set a goal and decide on the milestones to achieve that goal. If you miss any of the milestones, you can feel sad and/or anxious. If you miss the goal itself, then you can feel lost and stressed.

In reality, you may have an ultimate goal in life but it'll take at least 100 goals to achieve that goal.

Your ultimate goal is probably to "Be happy in life". Your other goals to achieve this ultimate goal could be:

1. Sustaining good health.
2. Having a debt-free house.
3. Having a happy family.

And so on.

You need to have milestones for each of these goals and try to achieve these goals. The beauty of having more than one goal is that even if you miss one goal, some other goal will compensate for it and help towards achieving your ultimate goal.

It's like playing the board game Mahjong. When you play Mahjong your ultimate goal is to win the game. But you need to achieve many smaller goals, like creating a strait or pairs, which ultimately contribute to the final win.

Who is lucky?

Alan was in his final year of an MBA. A Fortune-500 automobile company came to the campus on a recruitment drive. Considering Alan's background—he came from a typical middle-class family, and his father had to struggle to support Alan's education—this job would have been a dream come true for Alan. Alan cleared the first round of interviews and was selected as one of twenty shortlisted candidates for the second round. Alan's hope for the highly paid job increased and his plans for spending the money had already begun. Alan prayed to God that he would clear the rest of the rounds and get the job. To his pleasant surprise, he cleared the second round and was selected for the final interview. Now it was a do or die situation for him. He had to do his best to clear the final round as it was the last milestone to land the job. During the final round of interviews, Alan was desperate in his efforts to get the job, but somehow he did not succeed. His classmate was selected for the job instead. Alan felt as though everything was over. He spent a couple of days drinking and smoking cigarettes. It took a while for him to recover from the sadness he felt. He finally collected himself and put his efforts into finding another job. Getting a job was important to him as he'd spent twenty-four years of his life getting the education, and now it was time to not rely on his father's financial support.

Alan managed to get a job. It was not highly paid but at least he had a job. That year, recession hit the world and almost half of his classmates were struggling to find a job. So Alan felt lucky. After spending six months in the job, Alan was being bullied by one of his colleagues in the office and he started feeling that he was unlucky working there and having these kinds of colleagues. Alan started his job search and landed a role in a bigger organisation and with a better salary. Alan felt lucky again. The new organisation was growing at a rapid pace. Alan enjoyed the new work and the company of his new colleagues. After a few months, the company had a few big international projects on the go. These involved international travel and exposure. Alan did not get the opportunity to work on these projects. So he felt unlucky and became sad. His colleagues left for international travel but the plane they were travelling on met with an accident. No one survived. Alan felt lucky. Alan got another job that did involve international travel and he felt lucky again.

One thing Alan finally realised is that there is nothing called lucky or unlucky. Things happen. And there are always ups and downs. If you get something you want that's great—celebrate the achievement and be happy that you achieved it—but if you don't get something you want, *it is still okay*; something else might be on its way to make you happy.

They say choose the manager, not the company, as people leave managers not the company. When you are joining an organisation, you have the freedom the join the manager.

Unfortunately, these days, status doesn't remain the same for long in any organisation as a result of constant restructuring. You may feel lucky if you join a manager you like and unlucky if you join a manager you don't like. But nothing remains constant. Chuck the concept of lucky and unlucky away, and embrace the ups and downs.

Existing problems cannot always be solved by the current level of thinking

If you don't solve a problem in time, it may have a severe effect.

There used to live a happy monkey in a village. The whole day, he jumped from tree to tree, plucking ripe fruits and eating them. The village also produced plenty of nuts. Villagers used to store the nuts in big baskets before dispatching them for sale. Nuts were the monkey's favourite food and he had no difficulty in accessing them. So life was happy for him.

One day, the monkey went out to grab some nuts. But this time there was something unusual. The nuts were stored in a jar. Monkey put his hand into the jar, made a fist with the nuts inside his hand, but because the opening of the jar was narrower, he could not pull out his hand. Going back without the nuts was difficult for the monkey. He tried many times but in vain. His efforts made some noise, which was heard by the villagers. Soon the villagers came with their sticks and beat the monkey. The monkey was beaten almost to death, but somehow he managed to escape.

This is a classic example of a problem where we think there is only one solution or no solution at all.

The monkey decided to never eat nuts again in its life.

A few days later, the monkey got some company. The new monkey made the same mistake of putting its hand into the jar, but soon realised it was not going to work. He picked up the jar and ran into a jungle with it, poured all the nuts on the ground and enjoyed them.

We come across similar situations in an office environment. If a problem is not addressed on time, a small problem can blow out of all proportion and threaten the jobs survival of the employees. So it is important to make your mind ready to think beyond the level of the traditional problem-solving approach.

The need to go beyond motivational talk

Sometimes when we feel low, a motivational talk can come to our rescue. A motivational talk can help to release feel-good hormones and we feel happy. The corporate world uses motivational talks to bring about change, make employees feel good about their roles and the organisation.

The only drawback of motivational talks is that they have a short-term effect. It's like drinking a coffee when we feel low. Caffeine gives us a kick and stimulates the brain and we feel better, energised and excited. But the effect remains only for a few hours and then we come back to the original situation after the caffeine has worn off. When we watch a movie and heroic acts we feel motivated. After watching a movie, we also feel excited and feel like we also may have those heroic qualities. But after some time we come back to earth and realise we are just normal human beings and we cannot perform those heroic acts.

Similarly, when we hear motivational talks we feel good and motivated. We feel like we can do anything. This effect may remain for a few days, even a few weeks. After some time, however, the talk becomes a memory and fades into the big storehouse called the mind. You may keep retrieving it for some time but then, eventually, it is lost in the storehouse. Whether it's coffee or a motivational talk, both are external and we are dependent on that. Both are addictive. That's why there is a need to have something of our own that we can use whenever we need to, to make us feel good and happy. We need something similar to caffeine that flows in the blood to make us feel good. We need something similar to a motivational talk that will stimulate the mind and make us feel happy.

Stress management... Really?

You manage things that are present all the time; for example, your blood pressure. You need to manage things that are not reversible. Do you manage the problem or solve it? If stress is the problem, you need to not manage it, you need to solve it.

Do you know that the term "stress" did not exist before 1935? In 1930, a scientist named Hans Selye conducted an experiment on mice. He injected mice with different irritating substances, subjected them to extreme conditions, such as temperature and noise, and found that the response was the same—swelling on certain parts of the body, heart attack, kidney failure, etc. He found that there was a similar correlation for humans between the situation and the response. Humans show a similar pattern when they find themselves frustrated and exposed to constant discomfort. So the term was coined as "stress". Stress is a response to events. The response comes from what we perceive and experience. Handling stress is about controlling the response. Unless we go to the root of how we respond, we won't be able to remove the stress. The response could become a habit and we might keep responding in a similar way to major as well as minor events.

Stress needs to be *removed* not managed.

If we need to address a problem, we need to understand its root cause. If we need to remove stress, we need to understand what the root causes of our stress are.

The main external causes of stress are:

- FOMO—fear of missing out
- insulting words
- the pain of separation from loved ones
- the pain of losing wealth
- fear of losing health.

Stress needs not to be managed; its root causes need to be managed.

When we look at the root causes of our stress, the search usually ends with the people and things around us. For example, people's behaviour, or things we don't have or can't achieve. Going a little deeper, if we try to find where this stress originates, we will reach into our own mind. Surprisingly, our own mind is the internal root cause of stress. The mind interprets behaviour, which leads to stress. We need to fix or control our own mind to reduce stress, rather than trying to control people or things around us that are external factors.

There is only one who can be our biggest foe or greatest friend— our own mind. Once we convince our mind to be our friend, we don't need to think about stress. Yogic life gives the utmost importance to the mind and its functioning.

Pareto principle

The Pareto principle, also known as the 80/20 rule, is named after scientist Wilfredo Pareto and focuses on a vital few rather than the trivial many things or factors. According to the principle, all things in life are not always evenly distributed. The principle was originally used to describe the uneven distribution of wealth. It says that twenty percent of the people have eighty percent of the wealth. It stands true in today's world as well. When we look around us, roughly twenty percent of the countries have eighty percent of the wealth. Similarly, within a country, roughly twenty percent of the people are the richest and have eighty percent of the total wealth of the country.

The Pareto principle is important to understand because many aspects of our life follow the same principle:

- Twenty percent of things consume eighty percent of your income.
- Twenty percent of activities take eighty percent of your time.
- Twenty percent of people cause eighty percent of problems.

Similarly, twenty percent of the causes are responsible for eighty percent of the problems in our lives.

The Pareto principle is simple and it suggests that focusing on a vital few problems will take care of a maximum portion of the response, leaving behind the trivial many to address later.

We get stuck into so many trivial aspects of life that we ignore important aspects. If we use the same principle to stress, then twenty percent of things will cause eighty percent of the stress in our life. The goal is to identify that twenty percent and manage it well.

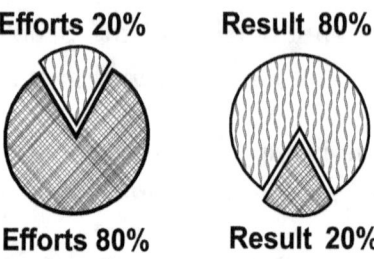

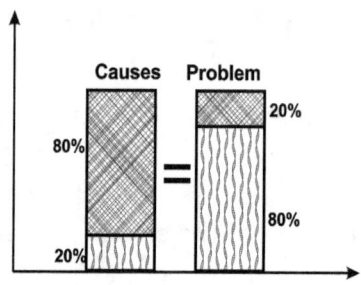

Fig.-Pareto Principle

Cut the garbage

GIGO—Garbage in, garbage out.

What you take in decides the quality of what you process and what you produce.

This terminology is commonly used in the software industry, and means that if the wrong information is fed to software, we will get the wrong output. It is applicable to the human body as well. If we eat the wrong food, we will get the wrong effects. If we inhale the wrong air (contaminated or polluted), we get the wrong output (we get sick). The third thing, which is invisible but

54

works in the same way, is that what goes into our mind creates the effects accordingly. The mind gets inputs from what we see, read and hear and produces output in terms of behaviour. Negative talk makes us feel negative, while positive talk makes us feel positive. We cry if we see tragedy on screen because the mind is reacting accordingly.

In many cases, the mind can't differentiate what is real and what is fake. When we use negative words, we also feed negative information to our mind, so it is important that we always try to speak positively. While what we speak is in our hands, it is difficult to control what others will say, do or show you. So the best thing is to make the mind not be affected by these external factors. The way exercise makes the body stronger and more able to face external attacks, similarly, yoga and meditation can make the mind stronger and less susceptible to negative thoughts or the environment around us.

Your mind plays back what you feed to your mind. So if people are talking negatively, you need to learn to stop being fed by those thoughts. See the difference.

I remember being on a road trip in Australia. Just like any typical road trip, it had been planned hastily and the only thing my work colleague and I made sure of was that we had music and food with us. We left after the office closed so it was already late. A couple of hours later, we'd probably spent more time on taking breaks than on the road. After another three to four hours, we decided to stop somewhere and camp. My friend found a campsite and we followed the direction on the map. It was a secluded place, and when we got out of the car, no one else was around. This isn't common in summer in Australia as most campsites are crowded in this season. We were discussing whether it was actually a campsite or a private property because we were worried about fines for illegal camping.

The area looked good though so we felt comfortable to camp there. Suddenly, my friend noticed a sign that read "graveyard". We realised the GPS had landed us in a graveyard. Immediately after realising this, my friend said he could smell flesh. That was weird because the place felt fresh before we read the sign, and now suddenly we had the smell of flesh! Anyway, we immediately left, of course. After checking the GPS carefully, we realised that the campsite was on top of the hill and we had gone to the bottom of the hill. We steered our car and reached the right place.

That's how the mind plays the game: it interprets based on what information it is given.

Joy and pleasure

Pleasure comes from the external activities we do, whereas happiness and *joy* come from within. Joy does not exist in the materialistic world; it exists within the heart.

Generally, what upsets us is everyday life trivia, such as being pressurised by the boss, bullied by colleagues, having a fight with our spouse or failing an exam. All these little things that happen to us throw us off balance.

Pain and pleasure are the inherent nature of four psychic instruments: the mind, subconscious mind, intellect and ego. They come and go. Pleasure becomes pain and pain becomes a pleasure. When you eat lots of sweet foods, it may give you pleasure, but its result—diabetes—may give you lots of pain. When you study for an exam, it may give lots of pain, but the result may give pleasure. This is a cycle. What is missing in this cycle is the *joy* of living life.

Joy is always in the present. It cannot be planned in the future. Joy will always lead to pleasure.

We put ourselves in pain in search of happiness.

It was a Monday. I had reached the office, checked my emails and was about to go for a coffee. A message came through on the communicator: "Ravi, I want to talk to you." If you get this kind of message on a Monday morning, it means something is not right.

This message came from one of my colleagues. We both came from same the city (Mumbai in India), so we had kind of bonded like siblings. At that time our organisation was going through a lot of restructuring and, as a result, many people were being made redundant. We were discussing this topic almost every day over lunch, and my colleague was particularly worried because she was fifty-plus in age. Her worry was that if she lost the job, she might not be able to get a new one. I had tried my best to motivate her to face the worst.

She had left India with her husband for better opportunities when they were in their thirties. They spent a few years in Singapore where they were blessed with a baby boy. After the birth of the boy, their whole world was focused around their child. For his better future, they moved to New Zealand. The kid grew up in New Zealand and got a good education. After his graduation, he landed a good job. By then, the parents had reached their fifties. They decided to move and settle in Australia to spend their retirement and live the unlived life, as their son wanted to go to the United States for further studies. They moved to Australia and started working there. It took them a couple of years to buy a house and feel settled.

After receiving the message, I immediately called my friend into a quiet room. Mentally I was ready to hear that she had lost her job so I was ready with my pep talk. As soon as she came into the room, she started crying. I knew something had gone wrong. So I tried to ask her. But she took a couple of minutes to stop crying. The only thing she had managed to say was "no" to all the questions I asked, like have you lost your job? Did someone shout at you? My thinking could go only to that level. She finally took a long breath and said, "My husband has been diagnosed with lung cancer."

I felt a deadly silence in my head. Before I could say anything, tears started rolling out of my eyes. It was a shock for me. I couldn't say a single word. I took a couple of minutes to open my mouth before I asked her questions: how, when, etc.? During these couple of moments, her life went through my mind. Both husband and wife had spent the whole of their life just focusing on their son. They hadn't even taken a proper vacation in their entire life. First, they were focused on raising the child, then his education and now they were thinking of his marriage, and then they just wanted to live their life, spend time with each other, travel, etc.

And they'd received this news. They had spent their entire life waiting for the right time to enjoy their life. The moment they felt that now was the time, it was too late. Time had gone.

My friend lost her husband after just a couple of months. She was in such shock that her health also started deteriorating. Both of them spent their life waiting for a perfect moment, which never came.

There is no perfect moment to be happy. It is now or never.

We are afraid to die because we are afraid that we have not lived. The more we move away from the real us, the more we stop living the way we want. In reality, you could be a writer, but work pressures do not allow you to be a writer. And you get the feeling of being lost.

If we want to transform ourselves, we need to purify our mind. A pure mind is a harmonious mind. When mind, body and soul coordinate, then the little upsets of the day can pass us by.

Who am I?

Ask this question of yourself. Keep asking this question until you run out of answers. Think of all the answers you have given. You will realise that none of the answers are permanent and your identity can change at any moment. That identity is true at that point in time only. For example, if you say, "I am a manager in a big organisation," you may have a completely different designation at the same time the next year. You may take your name as who you are, but you may be called by some other name by your friends, relatives or whoever. No identity is permanent. It's like when a cricketer is part of a cricket team for his country, then he will be identified accordingly. In India, there is the T20 cricket format. A team is formed by selecting cricketers from all over the world. A cricketer who is part of a team when he plays for his own country, may play against his teammates by becoming part of a different team. It's just like roles in movies. An actor who plays the role of a hero may play the role of a villain in their next movie. Life is like a play; don't take these identities seriously because none of them are permanent. Perform your duties diligently whatever role you're playing in the present, but don't let these roles destroy your inner peace.

Where are we going wrong?

Many times in our life we feel that things are going wrong. We struggle to understand why certain things happen to us.

Everything that happens to us can be attributed to the three Ps of consciousness, which are:

1. **Perceive**: understanding and selecting information from what we see and hear. We gather information in a conscious state (when we are awake). When we are asleep, we can't gather information and that is why it is similar to the unconscious state.

2. **Process**: planning and taking actions and decisions based on the information gathered. Everything we do needs some kind of planning and decision. Even the simplest task, like talking, involves planning and deciding what to say and what not to say. We store the information in our memory and use it to make decisions by processing that information. For example, when you drive a car, you know exactly how to drive the car because you have learned it before. You just process that information and make decisions accordingly.

3. **Prioritise**: becoming aware of yourself and your surroundings. Taking decisions based on information and events is not always sufficient; many times, things need

to be prioritised. A response to one event needs to be given over other events. For example, when you're eating a meal and the doorbell rings, you prioritise opening the door over eating your meal.

Fluctuation of the mind is the result of the imbalance of one or more "P" of consciousness. The importance of the above aspects cannot be underestimated. If the wrong knowledge is absorbed, it can lead to all sorts of wrong decisions. The second P, process, also involves imagination, but this can work for our benefit as well as against us. Imagination has to be accompanied by action to complete the process. The difference between imagination and action can also cause imbalance. For example, a product manager may imagine a new product, but unless it is manufactured, imagination has no value. Imagination is also treated as the future or a dream. Imagination makes you live in the future, depriving you of the present moment. Memory also has two aspects: damaging and liberating. Sad memories bring pain while good memories bring joy. Memory is past and can make you live in the past, depriving you of the present moment. Imagination is the future and memory is the past, while the present is in between them. Imagination and memory can cause an imbalance in the present.

"Those who fail to emerge from solely imaginative thoughts never command respect."

The goal of a student of yoga is to transform imagination and the past into the present with a positive state of mind while awake.

Happiness thieves

There are five thieves that steal our happiness. Interestingly, these thieves reside in our body. They are our five senses:

1. Touch
2. Sight
3. Hearing
4. Smell
5. Taste

The five sense organs are the conduit in the theft: the skin, eyes, ears, nose and tongue. These five sense organs act as the horses of a coach, called the mind. Imagine five horses pulling a coach in five different directions. It disturbs the functioning of the other organs as well as the mind. The mind gets pushed and pulled by the hunger of these sense organs, which creates imbalance—negative emotions such as stress and fear. A coach has to move, that is its objective, and horses have to pull it else we don't need the horses. The aim is to make the horses move in one direction, as the mind wants. When horses try to control the movement of the coach it causes chaos, but when the coach (with the help of a coachperson) controls the movement of horses, it moves smoothly.

Similarly, sense organs should not control the mind; the mind should control the senses. Controlling senses does not mean depriving them of their experience, it means letting them enjoy as much as is needed. For example, you might want to watch a TV series and finish the whole series in one go, but that greediness may cause strain on your eyes and other parts of your body. So your mind should control your eyes to make sure that your eyes do not spend excess time in front of the screen, resulting in strain.

WIIFM to WIIFU—a journey

Team members don't leave their manager when they feel that their manager is protective. It gives them the confidence to work without fear. Such teams have been proven as more effective. On the contrary, when a manager doesn't trust their own team members, it has been observed that such teams are the most disengaged. In this scenario, team members do not see any value in the work they do, they are not able to make decisions because of fear of punishment, and they engage in gossiping and making sure they don't lose their job. The team will be highly unproductive. In most of these scenarios, such a manager is of the view, "What's in it for me (WIIFM)?"

Why do they say that you should choose a manager not the company, or that you don't leave the organisation but leave the manager? Your manager helps decides how your life is going to be; happy/sad. When the manager just focuses on WIIFM, they are self-centric and won't care for anyone else. A good manager will always focus on what's in it for you (WIIFU). A manager who focuses on WIIFU can match the organisational goals with the individual goals of their team member, creating the win–win situation for the team as well as the organisation.

The journey is not about sacrificing what you want as an individual but to expand the sense of need for the whole team and, ultimately, for the whole organisation.

Where do you live?

"Why do you stay in prison when the door is wide open?"

—Rumi

We earn money and often one of the objectives is to buy our own house. Owning a house is most people's dream. An apartment, townhouse, house, villa, bungalow, whatever. There is often a desire to upgrade to a better place, too, as we think that home is where we spend most of our time. We also spend a lot of time at our workplaces. In reality, however, most of the time we live in our heads.

Even when we are at home, we keep thinking, dreaming, planning, remembering and contemplating—that's when we live in our heads. The same is true no matter where we are, whether we are on a train, on a flight or in our workplace; physically we are there but we still live in our heads and, sometimes, it can make us completely forget the world around us. Yogic life is about making the mind free of clutter and going deep inside the mind, taking shelter in calmness to stay away from all the trivial things that disturb us.

We try to maintain our physical property; we try to keep it clean and tidy. We know that a house with mess doesn't make us feel good. We try to have good light, air, fragrances, artefacts and plants in the house so that we feel good. The same is true for our heads. As we spend the maximum time in our heads, it becomes more important to maintain this place. We have to make sure:

- it is clean and free of rubbish (e.g., we get rid of negative thoughts)
- enough fresh light comes in (what we imagine)
- there are artefacts that make us happy (good thoughts).

If we don't pay attention to what is there in our head, that's when we start damaging the beautiful place with anxiety, stress, fear, etc. Healing is all about maintaining our headspace and getting rid of all negative aspects of life.

The following ideas can help to maintain our headspace or mind so that we have a beautiful place where we spend the maximum time of our life.

New turns vs wrong turns

When we shake the dice and throw it, we don't know what number we will get. We don't stop playing the game if we get a small number as there is still a chance of getting a higher number in the next throw. When the universe created us, we were not created to live in misery. You get up in the morning and start thinking about that unwanted phone call you received the previous day, and how it made you sad. You think about your broken relationship. You think about that lost opportunity... and you plan to live the rest of the day in misery. Just like getting a number on the dice, it can feel like a game of chance that we can't control; we can't control the events that are happening to us. We can't control the sunrise and sunset. We can't control the change in weather and natural calamities. We can't control the things happening around us. What we can control, however, is how we respond to those events.

When the sun rises we may feel lazy and we don't feel like going into the office because it feels like a toxic environment. What we miss out on is the opportunity to live another beautiful day. A small number on a dice is just an event, which will change in the next throw. Perhaps an event happens and we feel it's the wrong turn in our life. The feeling of the wrong turn can make the rest of the journey painful. A change in our response, however, and we could consider the turn as a new turn that will make the same journey exciting.

It's all about changing our perception towards things happening around us. Change of perception doesn't come with a cluttered mind. The mind needs to be calm and quiet and it will automatically do wonders.

"There are no wrong turns; there are only new turns."

Mind full to mindful

A cricketer may score a century in a match. But when they go to play their next match it's a completely new situation. It could be a different location, different time of day, different opponent, etc. The strategies they used to score 100 in the previous match may not be useful in the new match. What a successful cricketer does is analyse the situation in the new match and use the information and experience from previous matches to replicate the success. When playing, they have to be aware of the surroundings. A batsperson needs to be aware of the position of the fielders, their own position in the field, the way they hold the bat, etc. With all this awareness, they have to hit the ball with the right force in the right direction. You lose attention to one of these details and you may lose a point in the game. The chances of losing attention are higher if your mind is cluttered and you're not aware of the situation around you. If the player keeps thinking "success" or "failure" from the previous match, their mind will be full of thoughts, but instead they must focus on the situation around them at that moment; that is mindfulness.

There is a posture in yoga called the tree pose. It is one of the best poses to practise mindfulness. You need to stand straight and then bend one knee and place the foot of the bent leg on the inner side of the thigh of the standing leg. Then you raise both of your hands into a prayer or namaste position above your head. For a beginner, standing on one leg itself is difficult. After some practice, you can easily stand on one leg with the other leg bent and stay in the pose for longer. The real fun is the moment when you close your eyes—you lose your balance. Standing in the pose with your eyes closed takes lots of practice. An important aspect to be successful in doing this asana is to be mindful. The better you get at the pose, the more you become capable of being mindful whenever needed.

Stakeholder management

We can't please everyone.

Trying to please everyone is what we consider as stakeholder management. In most roles that are performed in a corporate environment, we have to deal with many stakeholders at a time. Organisations make things more complex when they introduce additional processes, such as dotted reporting or matrix structures. A flat organisational structure has an advantage over a hierarchical one as it reduces the number of stakeholders. While we can't control the behaviour of every stakeholder, what we can control is our own behaviour. You can't make everyone happy, but this doesn't mean that we have to make ourselves unhappy.

When we link our happiness with their happiness, that's where the trouble starts. Every day there will be at least one stakeholder who will be unhappy, so it means we will never be happy. If you count the number of times you are happy throughout the day, you will be surprised by the answer. That's why it's important to de-link our happiness with stakeholders' happiness. It doesn't mean not meeting their expectations. What it means is doing our best but not letting their behaviour spoil our happiness. Just like our body has an immune system to fight against harmful bacteria, so we need to have a similar immune system to prevent external unhappiness from entering our mind and impacting our internal happiness. Our body already has this mechanism; we just need to make it stronger so that we can handle all types of difficult stakeholders.

When you're looking for some information, and someone introduces you to a colleague and you think, ah that's the area where I wanted some information and I found the right person, you feel it's a coincidence. Whatever word you use to describe this situation, you can relate to the incident because your mind was looking for something. Whenever your mind is looking for something, you will get some clues or find that something. That's the basis of any discovery or invention.

If you're looking for love, you may find it in abundance the moment you start looking for it. But if your mind is agitated, you will see the whole world around you agitating. It's like closing your mind to love, so you won't see any evidence of love and will instead see everything that is opposite. It's a cycle. What you give will come back to you, and your response will trigger another wave of similar response back to you. You may come across some colleagues who never smile at you. That's okay. Just make sure about what you're sending—smile back. The next person may not smile back to you but at least it will leave an impression in his or her mind; his/her response will be with a little less ego. No one is looking for a bad, irritating response. Your smile can break the vicious circle.

No communication is 100% perfect

We see the world as per our senses. We believe that whatever our senses tell us is the ultimate truth. While watching a movie, we may cry when we see something sad happening on the screen. Our eyes and ears pass on the message to our brain about what appears to be the reality and the brain responds accordingly. When you're walking in the bush, if you hear some kind of slithering sound, you immediately hold your breath thinking it's a snake. In reality, it could be a big lizard. We come across so many such instances, and still we think that what appears is the ultimate truth. But what our senses communicate to our brain could be different to the reality.

As a kid, when I looked at a beautiful butterfly I would extend my figure towards it to let it know that it could come and sit on my finger. Most of the time the butterfly flew away, making me sad, and I never realised why the butterfly didn't listen to me. As an adult, when I play with dogs, I kind of face the same problem. I ask a dog to do something, but he doesn't necessarily do it. For example, I may ask him to sit down but he jumps around in joy. It makes me sad if he doesn't listen. In this situation, what I ignore is the basic process of communication. I expect the dog to understand what I say. When I ask him to sit, he may do so quickly after a lot of training. For me, I am asking him to sit but what I don't know for sure is what he understands, and I will never know. A pet will sync its behaviour to a certain extent with your communication, but we may never understand what the pet actually understands.

As human beings, we sync our behaviour with each other to a great extent. When I say good morning, you would understand what I mean by that. Many times, if you say something to someone, you know what you say, but the next person may not have the same understanding as you. If someone else says the same thing in a slightly different way, the other person may have a little better understanding. That's why, sometimes, if one professor teaches a subject, the students may not understand. The same subject taught by some other teacher may be well understood by the students. That's what we call a communication gap. What we communicate, we understand clearly, but the next person may not have the same understanding and may not respond to you as you expect. No communication is 100 percent perfect. It gets distorted, which gives rise to misunderstandings, differences and sore relationships. This impacts the corporate environment in a big way causing attrition, loss of productivity, office politics, and more.

Being mindful of the fact that no communication is 100 percent perfect will help to address many interpersonal issues.

A yogi understands that no communication is 100 percent perfect and, as a result, a yogi will be calm and quiet during turbulent situations.

Happiness pill

I went to a music festival in my teens and it was the first time I saw youngsters taking lots of drugs. The festival had a huge police presence, but still people had managed to get the drugs. I realised how common the use of drugs was when I saw so much of it during that festival. I saw many youngsters end up getting caught by the cops, hallucinating or experiencing a bad trip (a frightening and unpleasant experience triggered by psychoactive drugs, especially psychedelic drugs such as LSD and magic mushrooms). Those youngsters were taking drugs to feel happy, liberated, but in reality they were ending up with sadness and trouble. So the effect of those so-called magic-pills was definitely not happiness. It made me really sad and I never understood what they achieved by taking those drugs.

Most of the pills are made up of chemical substances that alter the chemicals in your body and brain. Most people take drugs to forget something and assume that the pill will bring happiness.

But there is another magic pill, which has been proven for thousands of years. It doesn't have any side effects but it creates effects on all aspects of your life. Yes, you can get addicted to it, and it can make you leave other addictions, too. It doesn't come in the form of a pill and you don't need to swallow it. It is called yoga and meditation.

Instead of a solid substance, you take air into your body in certain patterns, which helps to energise the body. These practices help to clear the clutter in the mind and help to wipe out unwanted memories. Once the mind is empty and the body is relaxed, the mind tends to attract positive thoughts, making us happy. Once you make it a regular practice, you become addicted to it. I have seen many people stop drinking after starting yoga and meditation as they don't see any value in the drinking anymore. Those who drink often say that one drink doesn't do anything, and if you drink a lot it does a lot of unexpected things as well. Then what's even the point of drinking? The same with smoking. Most of the smokers I know relate smoking with the state of their mind. If you are happy you smoke, if you are sad you smoke, and if nothing is happening, you smoke.

Once you are into yoga and meditation, however, when you are happy, you will do it, and when you are not happy you must do it. And if nothing is happening, you have to do it. If you have high blood pressure, you need to take a pill, even if you don't want to. Similarly, sometimes, even if you don't want to, you should still do yoga and meditation because it has similar effects to the blood pressure medicine. Things going wrong on the inside of the body can be corrected by sending the right substance into the body, which will keep the body in the right state—yoga and meditation.

When you take a medicine to manage a disease, it creates an impact inside your body. When you take drugs, drink or smoke, all these impact the inside of your body; for example, a psychedelic experience. Drinking and smoking also temporarily alter the state of consciousness, and that's why you don't see their effects for a long time. Similarly, yoga and meditation also create an impact inside your body.

Yoga and meditation are not for the external world but for the inward journey. If you focus on the external world, there are many other ways to showcase how good your body is, like through gymnastics or bodybuilding. You don't have to do yoga for that. The aim of yoga is an inward journey. You may buy a beautiful-looking mango, but if it's rotten from the inside, then that mango is of no use. Not every good-looking mango is good from the inside. Similarly, if a mango doesn't look good from the outside, we won't choose it. Yoga balances both. While it maintains the external appearance of the body, it equally helps to maintain the body from within as well. No other pill can do that.

Creating a rockpool

My friend Anna has three daughters. Separating from her husband was a big shock for her. She suffered domestic violence and also lost her house to her husband. When she received the news that she had breast cancer, she felt as though her world was over. Her beautiful daughters were two, four and seven at the time. She cried for days. Then she decided she had to be bold and fight against these odds in her life and try to be the strongest mum for her daughters. She believed that fight was for her life and that fight would keep her away from depression. Doctors fight diseases, soldiers fight enemies, police fight crime. Similarly, we have to fight against all the sorrows in our life. Fight keeps us away from depression.

Anna started her own café, and little hands accompanied her in her efforts. Her eldest daughter realised her mum's struggle and took responsibility for her siblings when necessary, and sometimes even helped take care of the café in her mum's absence, whenever she had to stay in hospital.

Anna has recovered now, but she still wants to prepare her daughters to fight every possible danger in life.

We all met in Newcastle recently for a picnic. Newcastle is a quiet little town two hours from Sydney and has beautiful beaches. We decided to take a swim before our lunch. Newcastle has a huge rockpool, and there is another rockpool inside the bigger rockpool. This smaller rockpool is great for kids as it's shallow. The eldest daughter, Celina, was looking a little sad because of something and wasn't enjoying the swimming; she was just looking at her younger siblings. Anna went and sat next to her. She picked up some small stones and started throwing them into the smaller rockpool. Every stone created a sound and ripples. After throwing three to four stones, she asked Celina to observe what was happening in the water. Again the same thing. Every stone made a sound and created a ripple. Then she said, "When we get sad news it's like getting hit by a stone in the water, isn't it? The event creates an unpleasant sound and affects us just like the ripples created by these stones. But look at these waves; they vanish after some time and even the stone that caused the whole ripple isn't visible. And did you notice that these ripples can't go beyond the boundaries of the pool? An unwanted situation in life is like a stone, and the water is like our mind. When this situation hits our mind, we get shocked, just like the stone makes a sound after hitting the surface of the water, and then just like the ripples we have after-effects of the incident, which are visible. But after some time, just like the waves disappear, our feelings disappear, too. So the skill is in how to make these waves disappear as soon as possible. Do you see the boundaries around the pool? A wave cannot go beyond the boundaries. If we create boundaries around our emotions, they cannot create longer effects. Even if there is an effect, it may be there for some time, but it won't expand beyond our boundaries."

The key to avoiding the bigger impact of the stone is to control how long its ripple can reach.

Who is superior: the fight of the five sense organs

One day, five sense organs of the body—nose, tongue, ear, eyes and skin—started fighting. Each sense felt that it was the most important for the body and kept arguing how the body would be useless without them. They kept arguing. No one was ready to accept that it was less important than the others. They decided to go to the mind to help them resolve the fight. Finally, the mind intervened and said, "Let's do an experiment. Each sense will leave the body for one day one after the other. The sense that has the worst impact on the body after leaving will be the most important." This experiment made sense to all the organs so they agreed to participate and prove their superiority over the others.

On the first day the tongue decided to take a break, leave the body and stop functioning. As per routine, the body went on eating but didn't taste anything. It was a horrible feeling. Whatever the body ate it was tasteless. The body couldn't differentiate between cold and hot, salty and bitter. The feeling was as if there was no meaning in eating anything. The body felt uncomfortable throughout the day and requested the tongue come back with the sense of taste the next day. The tongue was happy to have proved its importance.

On the second day the ears decided to take its break. The body stopped hearing. There was no sound at all. The body couldn't communicate with anyone, couldn't listen to music, watch

78

movies, etc. It disturbed the body because it started feeling lonely because of the lack of social interaction. The body requested the ears bring back the hearing sense the next day. The ears were happy to have proved their importance.

On the third day the skin decided to go on leave. It stopped sensing touch anywhere on the body. The body couldn't sense anything on the skin. It couldn't feel mosquito bites, while mosquitoes kept on sucking its blood. Its fingers couldn't feel the keyboard while typing. The hands couldn't feel anything while holding things, and it was difficult to understand whether the hands were actually holding stuff or not. The body stumbled throughout the day as the limbs couldn't function properly as they did not have any sense. The body got bruises all over it as it never realised when it was getting hit, and it became miserable. The body requested skin to bring back the senses the next day. The skin felt happy to have proved its importance.

On the fourth day the eyes decided to go on leave. When the body opened its eyes in the morning there was darkness everywhere. The body couldn't see anything. It was difficult for the body to even get out of bed and go to the toilet. The body became completely paralysed in the absence of eyesight. The body could not do any routine work throughout the day and had to be dependent on everyone else for almost every task. It was difficult to survive without seeing. The body pleaded with the eyes to come back. The eyes felt that they were most important among all because of the body's plea to come back.

The next day the nose went on leave. It stopped breathing. After a few seconds, the body started suffocating. After a minute, all the organs in the body became restless as they felt they were dying. All the sense organs also felt as if they were losing their sense. The mind also started feeling numb. The mind realised the consequences of not breathing and requested the nose to start breathing immediately. Nose agreed and started breathing. All organs and the mind felt relief. The rest of the sense organs and the mind went to the nose with folded hands and told nose it was the most important sense organ as it aided breathing. The body can live without the other sense organs for days, weeks, months and years, but the body cannot live without breathing even for a few minutes. All praised nose for its importance and unanimously declared nose as the king of all sense organs.

This hypothetical story supports the importance of the nose and its function, highlighting that breathing is the most important function.

Low energy to high energy

Food, water and air are three important elements for the survival of the human body.

How much do we eat every day? Roughly 2–3 kg.

How much do we drink? Roughly 2–3 litres.

How much air do we take in?

- We inhale roughly 500 mL per breath.
- On an average, we take 15 breaths per minute.
- We take 500 X 15= 7500 mL, i.e., 7.5 litres in a minute.
- 7.5 litres X 60 = 450 litres in an hour.
- 450 X 24 = 10,800 litres in a day.

So, our bodies consume more air compared to food and water. The body needs it. The question is, do we inhale the required amount of air throughout the day? We give the least importance to our breath. What do you do when you want to eat nice food? You go to a restaurant and spend hundreds of dollars making yourself happy. What do you do when you are thirsty or you want to drink a tasty drink? You won't hesitate to get a glass of water or spend money on drinks. How many times have you taken time out just to breathe and give your body enough breath? How many times do you take time out just to give your body pure air?

Breath helps to create energy. This energy flows throughout the body. Yogis call this energy prana. There are 100 nadis (nerves) in the heart. From each of these nadis, 72 branch out, and again each of these nadis has 1,000 sub-branches. Thus, there are 72 million nadis through which prana flows.

We get twenty percent of energy from food and eighty percent from breath. Our breath supplies oxygen to our body. Our body cells use the oxygen we breathe to get energy from the food we eat. The oxygen in our body is used to break down glucose and create the fuel for our muscles, called ATP. ATP, which stands for adenosine triphosphate, is the sole source of energy for all human metabolism, yet very little of this fuel is actually stored in the body. Cellular respiration is the process by which cells release energy from glucose and change it into a usable form called ATP. Cellular respiration uses oxygen to release energy for the working muscles. The energy is released in the form of ATP. When working muscle, our muscles have to work harder, which increases their demand for oxygen. When the body needs more energy as a result of the extra workload on the muscles; for example, from exercise, we breathe faster and supply the body with more oxygen to produce more energy.

So, oxygen-carrying molecules, such as haemoglobin and myoglobin, transport oxygen to where it is needed. The human body has roughly 37 trillion cells, out of which 27 trillion are red blood cells. Red blood cells act as a transporter of oxygen.

The body needs a certain amount of circulating oxygen in the blood at all times to effectively nourish the cells, tissues and organs. When blood oxygen levels drop below normal, a condition known as hypoxaemia may occur.

Low blood oxygen levels can result in abnormal circulation and cause the symptoms of:

- shortness of breath
- headache
- restlessness

- dizziness
- rapid breathing
- chest pain
- confusion
- high blood pressure.

One of the ways to ensure your blood is infused with oxygen is to regularly exercise. When you exercise, the cells in the body burn oxygen faster than the regular rate. As the carbon dioxide levels in the body increase, your brain increases the respiration rate to get more supply of oxygen. Your lungs and heart perform at optimum capacity during exercise to intake more oxygen. It has been observed that people suffering from COPD (chronic obstructive pulmonary disease), and the subsequent low-oxygen saturation, can enhance blood oxygen levels through exercise.

Benefits of better breathing:

1. Boosts your energy and stamina.
2. Counters tiredness and can lessen your need for sleep.
3. Relieves tension in your body and enhances your ability to deal with pressure and stress.
4. Brings a sheen of vitality to your complexion and eyes.
5. Boosts your immunity and releases chemicals that promote healing.
6. Increases your power of concentration and clear thinking.
7. Brings calmness and mastery to your emotions.

Better breathing also increases lung capacity; and the higher the better as more lung capacity means more energy.

Vital capacity is the maximum amount of air a person can expel from their lungs. People with a higher lung capacity will absorb more oxygen, resulting in more energy. So they will be more energetic compared to people with a lower lung capacity. Lung capacity is a key way of assessing people's fitness for the military and certain other occupations.

We suffer from the tomato effect

I am not referring to La Tomatina festival here or the effects of tomatoes on the human body. I am referring to the tomato effect as a habit rather than the effect of a physical phenomenon.

So what is this tomato effect?

The tomato effect refers to the belief in the 18th century in North America that tomatoes were poisonous because they're members of the nightshade family. I'm not kidding. Americans actually thought tomatoes were poisonous and never ate them. Even though the Americans knew that people in Europe had been eating tomatoes for more than 200 years, their common sense demanded that tomatoes not be eaten. This view of ignoring or rejecting experience because it does not make sense in light of popular beliefs or common understandings is called the "tomato effect".

Have you experienced the tomato effect? I feel it's so rampant; you can feel it everywhere.

When we know that helping each other in the office environment will create win–win situations, we still try to be individualistic.

When we know that yoga can make our life healthy, yet we hardly practise it.

And so on... if I keep listing instances, I will get tired!

Is there any sauce that can help me and everyone else to reduce this tomato effect?

Yes, there is. The answer is yogic life. Yogic practices are the panacea for all the pain, problems and questions.

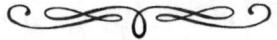

Chapter 2

Yoga—The journey

Yoga is a science where everything is based on matter and energy. The human body is made up of matter and energy, and yoga is all about balancing those well.

Yoga and meditation are not about becoming someone, but being the real us. Yoga is about living life fully but not to excess or addictively. If we can understand how our mind and heart work, we have the chance to answer many questions.

Yoga is not just about physical strength and flexibility. The goal of yoga is freedom from stress, anxiety, negativity, diseases, etc. There will still be pain in life, but yoga will give you the strength to bear the pain. No matter how big the pain is, you will forget about it during the journey. There will be questions that, sooner or later, we all end up asking ourselves such as, "Who am I?", "Why do I exist?", "Where am I going?" and "What should I do?" Yogic practices provide reasonable answers to such profound questions.

What most people want is the same. Most people simply want physical and mental strength, understanding and wisdom, peace and freedom. Yoga brings freedom. To a yogi, freedom is not being bothered by the dualities of life, its ups and downs, and its pleasures.

Yoga is like truth-bearing light, which helps to begin a new life. Old, unwanted impressions are discarded and we are protected from the damaging effects of new experiences. Yoga allows you to rediscover the wholeness in your life where you always try to bring different pieces together.

Power of thoughts

Your mind is like a storyteller. It keeps telling you the stories, but you need to tell your mind what stories you want to hear. If your mind tells you sad stories, this may lead to depression. A depressed person keeps on thinking about the same thoughts over and over again. Your emotions are the results of your thoughts.

The relationship between emotions and thoughts can be seen below:

- Fast and varied thinking results in elation.
- Fast and repetitive thoughts trigger anxiety.
- Slow, varied thinking leads to a sense of calm, peaceful happiness.

- Slow but repetitive thinking tends to sap energy and is said to spur depressive thoughts.

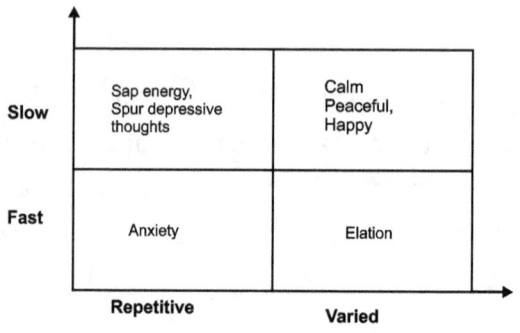

Fig.- Power of thoughts

The yogic journey is to move to slow and varied thoughts to remain calm, peaceful and happy.

Once the mastery over the speed and variation is achieved, then focus can be shifted to the quality of thoughts. Thoughts can be broadly divided into two types: thoughts that lead to action, and thoughts that do not lead to actions but produce a never-ending cycle of thoughts. The second type of thoughts do no good. Negative thoughts have more tendency to stay in the cycle. We are the best judge to decide which thoughts are good to lead us to action. Thoughts that don't lead to action but just speculation should be interrupted so as to avoid the cyclic nature.

Whenever you feel restless or unsettled, check what's happening with your thoughts. And try to slow down and not hold onto any thoughts. It will do wonders. Similarly, when you realise that you are breathing faster, just concentrate on your breathing and it will gradually slow down. Slowing down your breathing will reduce anxiety.

Five states of mind:

1. Kshipta—Disturbed
2. Mudha—Dull
3. Vikshipta—Distracted
4. Ekagra—One-pointed
5. Nirodhah—Mastered

The objective of the yogic practices is to master the mind.

Decide who you want to entertain

In olden days, many tribes did not have doors to their huts. The problem was that guests could come in and sit as long as they wanted. It was difficult to ask those guests not to come in because of social ties. The only way to avoid those guests was to stop entertaining them. Once the guest felt ignored, they used to leave on their own. Our mind is like those huts without doors, and the unwanted guests are those unwanted thoughts. If we keep entertaining those unwanted thoughts, they will stay there for longer, but the moment we ignore them they will go on their own. Once we start ignoring those unwanted thoughts, they may never come back.

Does every monk get a chance to sell his Ferrari?

Maslow's hierarchy of needs is one of the best-known theories of motivation. Humanist psychologist Abraham Maslow proposed this theory to describe the stages of growth in humans. The theory talks about self-actualisation as the topmost level in the hierarchy of human needs. Self-actualisation represents growth of an individual towards fulfilment of their highest needs; those for meaning in life, in particular. In Robin Sharma's famous book, *The Monk Who Sold His Ferrari*, the monk in discussion probably reached the self-actualisation stage and went to the Himalayas in search of peace.

But, yes, an important fact to notice is that this guy owned a Ferrari before selling it. How many of us will reach that level? Big question mark.

Out of curiosity, I Googled the names of people who have reached the self-actualisation stage. I was expecting a big list. After all, we live in a modern, high-tech world. To my great disappointment I found only a few names, such as Abraham Lincoln, Thomas Jefferson and Albert Einstein, who are considered to be people who reached the self-actualisation stage. We can easily find the list of the richest people in the world, but I had a tough time identifying the list of people who have reached the self-actualisation stage.

Is self-actualisation a myth? If not, how important is it? Can you achieve self-actualisation only if you become rich?

I looked again at Maslow's hierarchy.

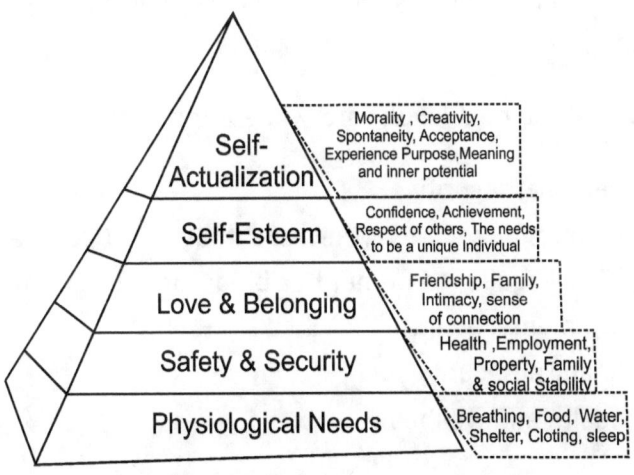

Fig.- Maslow's Hierarchy

Looking at the basic layer, physiological needs include:

- fresh air (breathing)
- water
- food
- sleep
- clothing
- shelter
- sex.

How many of us meet all these needs? How many of us breathe properly? How many of us drink enough water? How many of us eat the proper food and get enough sleep? And I started wondering, how many of us successfully cross this basic level?

I looked back at my education; my schooling, engineering and business management. None of these qualifications gave me a detailed understanding of these aspects.

Let's look at the next level. Safety needs include:

- personal security
- emotional security (they say that by 2020 the biggest killer is going to be neither blood pressure nor diabetes, but mental health)
- financial security
- health and wellbeing.

Same question: how many are crossing this level? This thought created doubt about Maslow's hierarchy in my mind. Then I read this statement, which addressed my confusion:

Maslow believed that to understand this level of need, the person must not only achieve the previous needs but master them.

Maslow's hierarchy is not a ladder to climb from one step to the next, but an overlap of needs to a great extent. Maslow probably directed us towards the solution, which we ignored in the fast pace of life:

Basic needs:

- Breathing properly—do breathing exercises, i.e., yoga and meditation.
- Water—drink enough water.

- Food—eat healthy food.
- Sleep—sleep well.
- Safety needs—take care of your personal safety.
- Emotional security—meditation.

I was reading about Maslow's hierarchy while I was on the train going to work early one morning. I looked around me. Most of the people were trying to catch a nap as if they had not got enough sleep during the night. Others were lost to their mobile phones. A couple were staring into space, and one or two were reading books. And I thought, how many of them are on a self-actualisation journey? If not, where are they going?

Yogic practices suggest that self-realisation can be achieved through consistent and rigorous practise of yoga by conquering the main obstacles to achieve happiness, such as desire, anger, greed, infatuation, pride and envy.

The self-realisation journey through the yogic way has three important components:

1. Balancing body
2. Balancing breath
3. Balancing mind

Control over these three aspects helps to achieve self-realisation. Control over each of these aspects brings immense joy and health benefits.

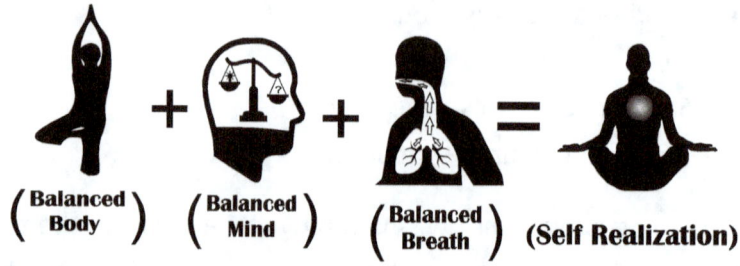

$$\left(\begin{array}{c}\text{Balanced}\\\text{Body}\end{array}\right) + \left(\begin{array}{c}\text{Balanced}\\\text{Mind}\end{array}\right) + \left(\begin{array}{c}\text{Balanced}\\\text{Breath}\end{array}\right) = \text{(Self Realization)}$$

Fig.- Self realization

The current definition of a yogi is someone who can demonstrate the yogic postures well. If you consider the yogic practices as an iceberg, postures are the tip of the iceberg. Very few make the effort to look at the whole iceberg, and therefore miss the yogic journey.

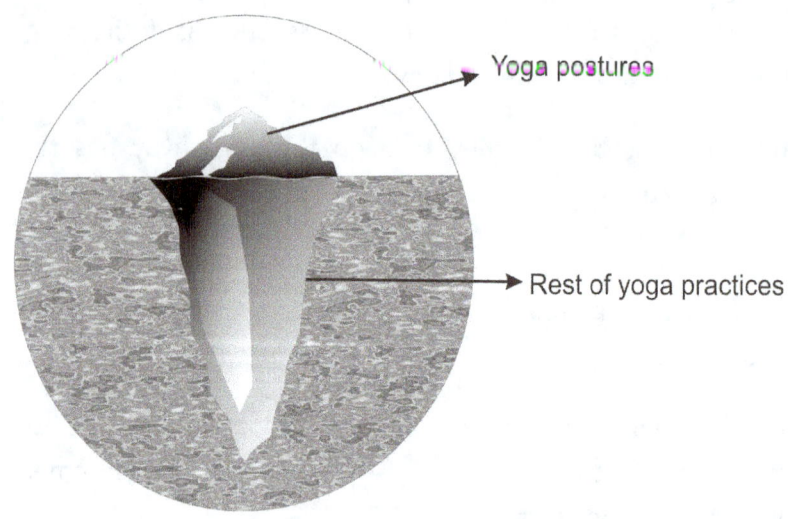

Fig. Iceberg of yoga

The yogic journey proposes practising eight aspects to achieve self-realisation:

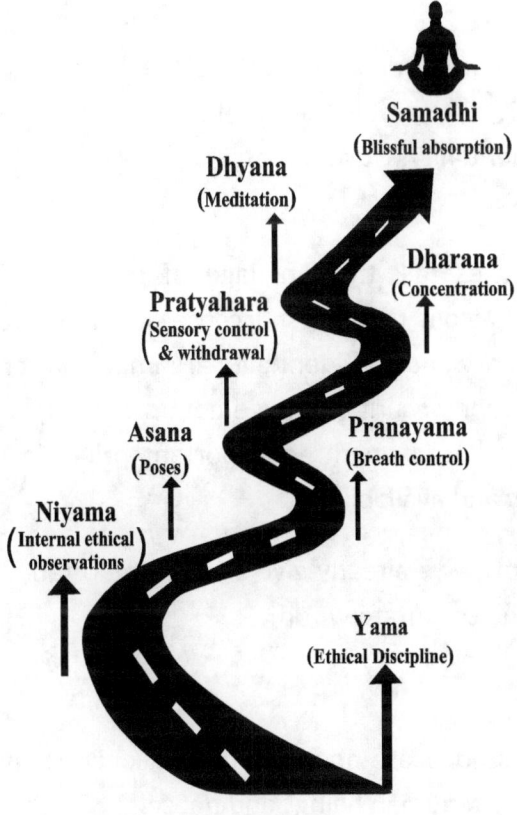

Fig.- Yogic Journey

Yama—ethical disciplines

Yama, or ethical disciplines, talks about principles of interaction with oneself and the rest of the world.

While yogic practices propose five different ethical disciplines, I find the following three the most relevant to the corporate world:

1. Nonviolence (no harm to others)
2. Integrity (no theft, honesty, etc.)
3. Confidentiality (trust, honesty)

Most HR policies talk the language of nonviolence; that is, promoting behaviour that doesn't cause any harm to others. In addition, integrity and confidentiality are important principles of ISMS (information security management standard). In fact, the whole ISMS is based on three important principles: integrity, confidentiality and availability.

So, inadvertently, we already give a lot of importance to ethical principles in the corporate world.

Nonviolence:

Yogic practices advocate nonviolence, not only against animals but against fellow human beings and oneself.

Vegan communities are a big advocate of nonviolence towards animals. Vegans refrain from using any type of animal products, such as milk, or things made from animal skins, like a belt or a drum. Vegan communities also do a wonderful job throughout the world creating awareness about animal cruelty. Veganism is based on the principle that every animal has an equal right to live and survive on this planet. Every animal has emotions, just like human beings. Animals follow the same lifecycle as humans; they mate, give birth, hunt for food, get old and die. Who are we to not let them live their life? Humans become selfish and abuse animals for their own benefits. Whether it's a newborn bird, piglet, baby seal, calf or a human baby—each is equally innocent and has an equal right to live. Taking their rights away by any means is violence.

Yogis treat all animals equally. In fact, the majority of places of worship have animals carved on the walls, symbolising equality. Yogis would never kill an animal to quench their hunger, and never keep a calf hungry to feed milk to their own children. Yogis use only those animal products that do not impact an animal in any way. For example, they may use a bird's dead feathers for decorating their room or to create a dream catcher. They may use the skin of an already dead animal to make clothes to protect themselves from the cold. But none of their actions would harm a living animal in any way.

Nonviolence against other human beings:

It's sad to see people killing people. Even wars can be won by not killing others. Mahatma Gandhi's nonviolence stance was against the British. Even though the British were brutal in suppressing the freedom movement, Gandhi decided to react with nonviolence against them. Wars are often fought based on geographical disputes, religion and natural resources. This makes no sense to me. Even when a geographical dispute has been addressed between two countries, the same issue still exists between regions in the same country, towns of the same region, and people living in the same town. What are we living for, dispute or peace? Since the time I was born, there has been some battle somewhere in the world with no end to the killing of millions of people. Those who kill, get killed eventually. But those who love, get loved. Surely that is a better way?

Violence is rampant in the corporate world, not in the form of direct killing or physical harm, but through mental harm. When employees are sexually harassed, or when managers bully team members, organisations create harmful work cultures. When you make others' life hell, it is still violence. You may not see physical symptoms but many suffer from mental disorders because of this violence, and many mental disorders lead to many tragedies. Stress is a major factor in diseases such as high blood pressure and diabetes, and organisations play a major role in imparting that stress to their employees. These diseases kill millions of people every year. Isn't that violence?

Asking or forcing your friends to drink excess alcohol or drugs is also a form of violence, as it is harming their body. Is your aim to take care of your friend or harm them? Ask that question when you're convincing them to drink or take drugs. There are hundreds of cases where youngsters die because of consuming illicit drugs just because their friends wanted them to do so.

Self-violence:

Torturing your own body is also violence. Torture doesn't mean burning your skin with a hot metal rod; it's any harm caused by you to your body. When you drink, use drugs, eat food that is not good for your body; this is violence against yourself as you're torturing your own body in a subtle way. The cruellest example of violence against self is committing suicide, and taking away your own right to live and survive.

Living a yogic life helps you to practise nonviolence against animals, against fellow humans, and against yourself. All these three aspects create a better environment for yourself and everyone around you. This first step itself brings a huge change in your life as you start believing more in love than hatred. You become more sensitive to the pain of others. All this will directly help you to maintain your own health, address family issues and address issues in the workplace with colleagues. Practising nonviolence will make your life happier.

If you practise nonviolence, it may not change the world, but it will definitely change your own world.

Niyama—internal ethical observations
"Without discipline, nothing can be achieved."

The five elements of Niyama are:

1. Cleanliness
2. Contentment

3. Discipline, austerities
4. Self-study
5. Surrender

Some of the benefits of practising Niyama are:

- Feeling of calmness, freshness, cheerfulness
- Fitness
- Mental comfort

You can't find answers in clutter

Whether it's your mind or the physical environment, you can't find what you want if it's untidy. The external environment and the mind go hand in hand. You can't expect a quiet mind among chaos. While yoga and meditation help to clean and calm the clutter inside the mind, we need to take efforts to maintain the external environment, too.

Immediately after finishing my engineering degree, I had an opportunity to work with a consultancy firm. My first assignment was to implement 5S, which is also known as a housekeeping philosophy in the manufacturing environment. It didn't make me happy initially. My impression (and so it is of others, and that's why you need consultants to implement 5S) about this philosophy was just to facilitate housekeeping. My mentor was a senior person who had spent all his life consulting manufacturing businesses. He understood my dilemma and he trained me in 5S. This changed my whole perception about this philosophy. Later, this became my ace card to show quick savings for many of my cost-reduction assignments.

5S is a Japanese methodology to manage inventory in a workplace (even though it's commonly recognised as a housekeeping principle, the term gives a slightly different perception about the philosophy). As the term suggests, the method has 5 "S"s, which are a roadmap to implement this methodology:

1. **Sort:** this phase suggests sorting things. For example, if you want to manage your workstation in a better way, sort everything on the workstation. There will be items that you use many times a day, once a day, once a week, once in a while, never, etc. Sort them accordingly.
2. **Set in order:** once you have sorted, arrange everything in order based on the need. This may involve removing items that you're not sure will ever be used. Arrange items depending on the frequency of use.
3. **Shine:** once you set everything in order, decorate the space and make it more attractive.
4. **Standardise:** this phase suggests "a place for everything, everything in its place". For example, a tool board in the garage.
5. **Sustain:** this is about the discipline of maintaining what has been achieved in the previous stages.

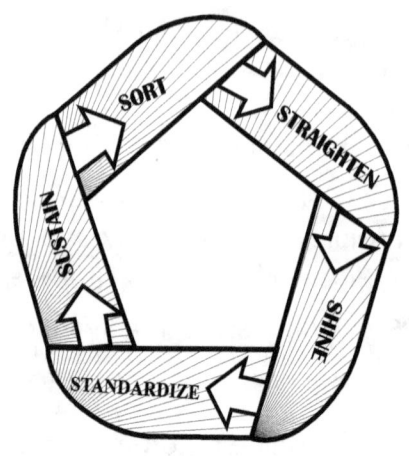

Fig.- 5S

This philosophy is so beneficial that almost every manufacturing plant uses it. There is also a concept of 5S that denotes the use of this practice in an office environment, such as for workstations, desktops, servers. It is equally beneficial to your house, laptop, garage, etc.

Practices such as 5S can help to clean and maintain the places around us, just as a shower will help to clean our body and yogic practices not only purify our body internally but also maintain them externally.

Postures—asanas

> *"Yogash chitta vritti nirodhah.*
> *Tada drashtuh svarupe avasthanam."*

Yoga is the mastery of the activities of the mind-field. Then the seer rests in its true nature.

-Patanjali Yog Sutra

Yoga asanas are normally called Hatha yoga. The meaning of hataha yoga is the sun (ha) and moon (tha). Yoga in which the sun is the soul and the moon is consciousness.

In yoga, the cause of a disease is the fluctuation of the mind. Asanas influence the chemical messages to and from the brain, which help to reduce the fluctuation of the mind, resulting in a healthy body. When we're engaged in a mental activity we're no longer aware of our body. Yogic poses integrate mind with body.

We have seven hundred muscles, three hundred joints, and sixteen thousand kilometres of nerve currents flowing through our systems, as well as 96,000 km of blood veins, arteries and capillaries. Regular practise of yoga asanas stimulates muscles, tissues, cells, relaxes joints and the nervous system and helps to maintain proper bloodflow throughout the body.

Fitness through yoga

Yoga does not receive as much attention as more physical exercise. The number of yoga studios is far less than the number of gyms. But total wellbeing (physical and mental) cannot be achieved just by putting pressure on our muscles. Exercise can be classified into two types: stimulative and irritative. If, at the end of the exercise, you or your body feels irritated, then you can classify that exercise as irritative, and if your body feels stimulated at the end of the exercise, you can call it a stimulative exercise.

Most physical exercises can be classified as irritative. When we think of physical exercise, it is all about gruelling workouts until we are exhausted. Lifting heavy weights, jogging longer and faster until our body says "no more please". Physical exercise solely focuses on making the muscles stronger. In reality, these types of exercises can do more damage to the body than good. They compress muscles, stiffen the joints, and acidify blood and tissues with excess lactic acid, carbon dioxide and other metabolic waste. Trained athletes make sure to deoxygenate the body by stretching and breathing, but most do not focus on that, leaving the body exhausted after exercise.

Yoga is a stimulative exercise. Body movements are harmonised with breath during yoga. It stimulates stagnated vital body fluids by massaging internal organs and glands and detoxifying them. It stimulates the movement of lymph. As lymph is involved in the purification of blood, proper movement of lymph through yoga helps to detoxify the body right to the cellular level. Yoga oxygenates and alkalises blood. It loosens the joints and relaxes muscles. This helps to increase the flexibility of the body. Yoga brings calmness, increases concentration and rejuvenates the whole body. It creates and stores energy instead of spending energy. It creates a perfect communication between each part of the body and mind. Yoga does not impact the external factors that create stress, but it gives mental strength to deal with stress and reduces the impact of stress on the body.

If you want to maintain the performance of your car, you will take good care of it. Speeding up the engine won't increase the performance of the engine, and driving longer won't make the tyres better. Excess use of the car means more wear and tear of the parts. Similarly, our body parts are subjected to wear and tear. Putting extra pressure or excess use on these parts can damage them. We need to be mindful of the right and optimum use of the body parts to increase their lifespan.

Purifying the body

When we wear clothes, they get dirty because of dirt, sweat, stains, etc. We clean the clothes in water and then squeeze the clothes to dry them. When we squeeze the clothes, water takes the dirt or other particles with it and makes the cloth clean again.

When our muscles get stressed, channels carrying energy in the body become blocked and toxins accumulate in various parts of the body. This requires a wash as well. Yoga helps to purify the body. When we do yoga we use breath to take the impurities out of the body. Hatha yoga focuses on physical postures. When we perform these, various organs in the body are squeezed, which helps to release the toxins accumulated in those organs. Yoga literally massages the internal organs of the body. Just like when we massage our body we press the body part and release it, which helps to relax the stressed muscles, yoga does the same thing to our internal organs. It squeezes and releases the organs, relaxing the various muscles of that organ.

Stressed or hard muscles always cause problems. Breath plays an important part in relaxing our muscles. Accumulation of lactic acid causes the muscle to spasm. This acid gets diluted when those muscles get enough oxygen, which is why, whenever there is muscle spasm, you get the advice to relax and take a deep breath and drink water. Drinking water also provides the body with additional oxygen. You've probably experienced muscle spasm at some point in time. That's how muscles become stressed and contracted, resulting in pain.

When athletes run they may suddenly get a cramp in their leg as a part of excessive pressure on their muscles. Massaging relieves the muscles from cramp. Similarly, when we are stressed, we get the advice to take a deep breath. Stress causes strain in various muscles of the body. Strained muscles can easily be experienced on our face. When you are angry or stressed, observe the contraction of facial tissues. We get similar effects on various tissues of the body when we are stressed. When we do yoga we supply the body with additional oxygen to relax those muscles. Yoga postures massage the stressed muscles and, as a result, we feel rejuvenated.

Art of balancing

Slackline is the art of balancing on a suspended length of webbing between two anchors—similar to tightrope walking. But how do you master it? The key for slackline is concentration and balance. When you are on the rope, even if you lose concentration for a fraction of a second, you lose your balance. When on a slackline, different forces influence your balance—bodyweight, wind, shakiness of the body, concentration, etc. When you lose balance you fall down.

Human life has many factors that try to imbalance it, such as family, health, career and aspirations. All these act like forces and try to pull you onto their side. It's important to maintain the balance, else we will fall down.

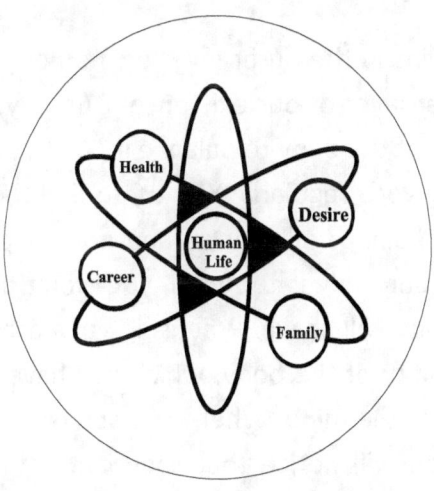

Fig.- Factors affecting human life

Yoga asanas are considered as the foundation of life. When you stretch your body and try to do an asana, you try to balance. When you are in an asana, you tend to look inward to your mind and body to try to create balance. For example, when you do the sun salutation (one of the most effective sequences of yoga postures), you stretch various parts of your body, and all your attention tends to come towards your external as well as the inner body.

Yoga asanas help to release tension in the muscles. When you are angry, you must have noticed that you squeeze your eyebrows, your throat becomes heavy, your eyes become smaller and you breathe rapidly. These are some visible symptoms. Similar impacts happen on many other parts of the body.

Relaxation begins in the outer layer of the body and penetrates into the deeper layer of our existence. During yoga asanas, you find the centre of the body to balance it. That becomes the habit after practising yoga regularly. You try to find the centre in your life as well, to balance all aspects and not get pulled by any of the forces. If your body is too rigid, you won't be able to do an asana. Your body will shake. Practising yoga asanas will help to reduce the rigidity of the body, which will have a direct impact on the rigidity of the mind. When a person is mentally disturbed or dejected you will notice that they can't stand properly on their own feet. These postures try to make the body stable, resulting in stability and calmness of the mind.

When you inhale, your body tenses, when you exhale, your body relaxes. Inhaling and exhaling along with the postures helps to supply extra oxygen to the internal organs involved in the posture.

Yoga and the Piezoelectric effect

The piezoelectric effect is the property of some materials to convert mechanical energy into electrical current. A piezoelectric substance is one that produces an electric charge when mechanical stress is applied (the substance is squeezed or stretched). Conversely, a mechanical deformation (the substance shrinks or expands) is produced when an electric field is applied. "Piezo" is a Greek word that means "to squeeze". "Piezoelectric" literally means electricity caused by pressure. The effect was first discovered by Pierre Curie and Jacques Curie in 1880.

In today's world of electronics, piezoelectricity is used everywhere. Asking Google for directions to a new location uses piezoelectricity in the microphone. There's even a subway in Tokyo that uses the power of human footsteps to power piezoelectric structures in the ground. Each time a passenger steps on the mats, a small vibration is triggered, which stores the energy.

You'll find piezoelectricity being used in many electronic applications.

Dr I. Yasuda, in 1957, discovered the existence of the piezoelectric effect in bones. Many researchers also believe that the whole human body is composed of materials arranged in a liquid crystal. Liquid crystals are "materials that are intermediate between solids and liquids and display properties of both". If our bodies can be considered as liquid crystals, and if even small movements create electric fields and currents, this could provide a basis for how yoga and massage might have an effect on the functioning of our bodies, and therefore on our health.

During yoga, our liquid crystalline tissues are subjected to deforming stress, which results in the generation of piezoelectric energy and tiny electric currents. A logical mind may think that the tiny electric currents may not have an effect on the body. Let's consider a metaphor of a mobile phone. Mobiles have a tiny chip, which acts based on a small electric current. That small electric current makes the mobile phone work. When you receive a call from your loved one saying he or she is safe after an earthquake, that small piece of information plays a big role in life. Similarly, when tissues are subjected to stress, small electric currents create a big effect on the body.

Yoga asanas can be broadly classified into the following:

- Forward bends
- Twists
- Standing
- Sitting

- Inversions
- Backbends
- Lying down

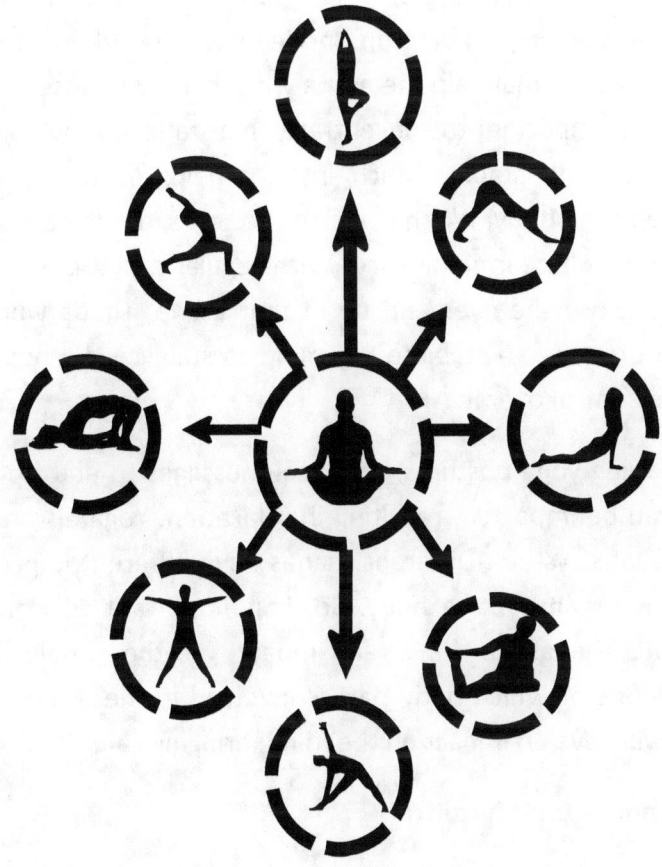

Fig.- Yoga Asanas

In every asana, you will observe that we need to identify the centre of the body so as to balance the body. Identifying the

111

exact centre is key for every asana. If the centre is not identified, we won't be able to attain the desired asana. When you identify the centre and get into the asana, your mind tends to concentrate. For example, when you are in the tree pose, described earlier (standing on one leg with the other leg bent), beginners can't maintain the asana with their eyes closed. In this asana, it is important to concentrate on a static nearby object to keep the mind stable, which in turn helps to maintain the balance of the body. When you close the eyes, the mind starts to deviate, resulting in imbalance. With regular practise, however, you can close the eyes and be in that asana. That's what the yogic journey is: to stabilise the mind to stabilise the body and achieve control over it.

While doing yoga postures, chemical messages to and from the body can be impacted, resulting in relaxation. Yoga also relaxes the nervous system. Different asanas have different impacts on different organs of the body. So, it is important to learn the different asanas to have an impact on the whole body. Irrespective of which body part is involved in the asana, every asana will have an impact on the mind, bringing calmness.

Pranayama—breath control

Our health and our existence depends on the breath. Respiratory function makes a breath part of the human body. Human life starts with the first breath as a newborn and ends with our last breath, accompanied by continued breathing in between.

Let's understand breath. To do so, we need to understand the respiratory system in the human body.

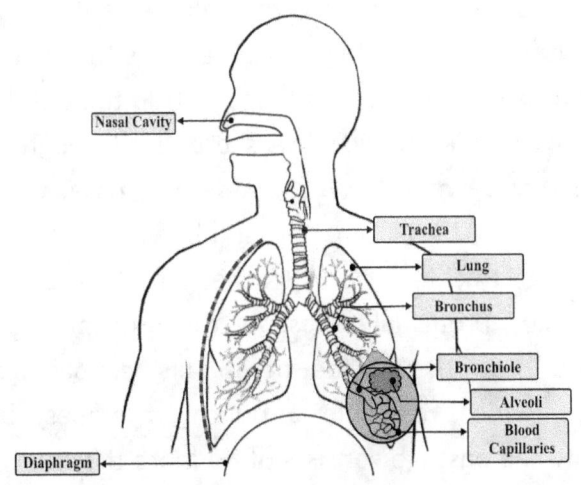

Fig.- Human respiratory system

Respiratory function stretches from our nose to the lungs. It serves two main purposes: bringing oxygen into the body through inhalation; and releasing carbon dioxide and waste matter through exhalation. As soon as you inhale, the respiration process begins. Inhaled air goes to the lungs, where gaseous exchange happens. Oxygen is absorbed into the bloodstream and carbon dioxide is released from the bloodstream. Oxygenated blood is then sent to the heart, which pumps the blood throughout the body, nourishing every organ with fresh oxygen.

The nose is the first part that is engaged in breathing. It acts as a filter to prevent foreign particles and bacteria from entering the body. The first line of defence is the hair inside the nose, which acts as a filter. The second line of defence is the sticky surface inside the nasal passage, which helps to trap the dust, bacteria, etc. That is why we should always breathe through our nose unless we require more oxygen. After the nasal passage, air passes through the back of the throat (pharynx and then through the windpipe, trachea). Your trachea then divides into air passages called bronchial tubes. As the bronchial tubes pass through the lungs, they divide into smaller air passages called bronchioles, which resemble a bunch of grapes, becoming smaller until the passage consists of no more than a single layer of cells. Each bronchiole ends in tiny balloon-like air sacs, called alveolus. Our body has over 300 million alveoli. The membrane enclosing each alveoli is surrounded by a mesh of tiny blood vessels, called capillaries. Here, oxygen from the inhaled air passes through the alveoli walls and into the blood. Blood then flows to the heart and the heart pumps the blood throughout the body. Oxygen in the cells is consumed by the cells, producing carbon dioxide, which is then carried to the lungs through blood and is then removed from the body when we exhale.

Every time you inhale, an equal amount of air is exhaled. The air we inhale comprises about seventy-eight percent nitrogen, twenty-one percent oxygen and one percent of other gases, including carbon dioxide. The air we exhale consists of the same level of nitrogen, but the oxygen level drops to fifteen to sixteen percent, while carbon dioxide levels go up to five to six percent.

Respiration is such a simple process of supplying oxygen to our body and throwing waste out of the body. Our lungs are always under constant threat from particles, chemicals and bacteria and are vulnerable to injuries and infections. Respiratory function-related diseases are increasing rapidly throughout the world. For example, chronic obstructive pulmonary disease (COPD) is the third leading cause of death throughout the world and it's increasing. The other most common diseases related to the respiratory system, and which are the most common causes of illness and death, are:

- asthma—a most common chronic disease of childhood
- acute lower respiratory tract infections, which take millions of lives every year (outbreaks of influenza add to these numbers)
- tuberculosis (TB)
- lung cancer.

Countries with high pollution levels are experiencing a rapid growth in lung disorders. The human body inhales polluted air and takes lethal substances into the body. This not only has an adverse impact on the respiratory organs but on the rest of the body as well, as these toxic substances get into the blood and the blood carries them throughout the body, damaging various parts of the body.

Smoking directly impacts the lungs and causes inflammation and irritation. The lungs should be in good condition to function properly. Smoking also destroys lung tissue and decreases the number of blood vessels in the lungs. Fewer blood vessels means reduced capacity to transport oxygen to the rest of the body. Less oxygen to the internal organs means we deprive them of oxygen, making them vulnerable to damage. A smoker feels stimulated after smoking, but that is a momentary effect. As their lung capacity reduces, their body starts feeling lethargic because of the decrease in oxygen. So, logically, it also impacts the functioning of the brain. Just as tooth decay starts with the accumulation of food particles and reaches a stage where the tooth needs to be extracted, organ decay starts with a reduced supply of oxygen and can suffer damage in different forms.

The haemoglobin in your red blood cells has 240 times greater infinity for the carbon monoxide you inhale from cigarette smoke than it has for oxygen. If you are a smoker, or if you live with a smoker, five to fifteen percent of your haemoglobin may be tied to carbon monoxide, even when you're not actually smoking. You then have less haemoglobin available to carry oxygen to the cells.

The most important thing required for the proper functioning of the brain is oxygen. Thousands of metres of minuscule capillaries pump hundreds of litres of blood to and from millions of neurons to maintain a constant supply of oxygen to the brain. The brain normally consumes twenty-five percent of the body's total metabolic energy, all of which depends upon the adequate supply of oxygen. Deficiency of oxygen can cause serious damage to the brain, which has unfortunately become a common condition throughout the world. Pranayama (breath control), on the other hand, enhances the practical cerebral function of the brain. Therefore, it is the brain that realises the most dramatic improvement in function that results from increased oxygenation of blood and tissues, and the improvement in microcirculation produced by pranayama.

In our day-to-day busy lives, we don't give the required oxygen to our bodies. There are two things that contribute to this:

1. **Blocked nostrils:** close one of your nostrils and breathe in and out from the open nostril. Now close the other nostril and breathe in and out from the open nostril. Most people will observe that one of their nostrils is a little blocked. Blocked nostrils means less flow of air through them.

2. **Shallow breathing:** when you're working in an office environment, stop doing everything for a moment and observe your breath. You will realise that you feel the flow of air in the front part of your nostrils only. Now, take a deep breath, and exhale. With a deep breath, you will feel the movement of your diaphragm and the flow of air deep in your nose and throat. That is what the body needs.

Apart from the above two factors, sleep disorders can cause reduced absorption of oxygen. People who snore at night often feel sluggish during the day. Snoring causes a reduced supply of oxygen to the body, resulting in lowered energy. Millions of people throughout the world suffer from sleep-disordered breathing.

Irregularity in the breath is another most neglected area that can contribute to breathing-related problems. Four major breathing irregularities are:

1. Jerks
2. Pauses
3. Shallowness
4. Noisiness

Ideally, there should be no jerks, no pauses, no shallow breaths, and no noise while breathing. The presence of one or more symptoms in your breath may be an indication of something not right, either with your breath, body or mind.

So, whatever loss of oxygen and its resulting impact on the body has happened during the day/night can be replenished by doing pranayama.

The breath helps to create energy. Ancient Indian yogis call it prana. It's called chi in Chinese and ki in Japanese. Prana is the energy in the body. Ayama is the creation, distribution and maintenance of it. So pranayama means creation, distribution and maintenance of energy. When you look at an electric cable, you can't see it but that doesn't mean that it doesn't have electric energy. If you touch it, you will feel the energy. Similarly, we can't see the prana in our body but it is there. You can feel it using many medical devices. If you stand below an electric cable carrying high-voltage electricity, you can hear the vibrations in the cable. Similarly, when energy flows through the body with high speed, you will feel the vibrations in various parts of your body, including your hands and face. It can easily be felt when you go for a run.

Art of Living founder, Sri Sri Ravi Shankar, has introduced a breathing method called "Sudarshan Kriya". When you do this rhythmic breathing as prescribed, you will feel the flow of prana throughout your body because of the flow of energy. Your breath directly contributes to the energy in your body.

Pranayama is systematic breathing. It has three parts:

1. Inhalation
2. Exhalation
3. Retention

There are different types of pranayama depending on the variation of these aspects. Pranayama techniques need to be learned from an expert because they have a direct impact on many vital internal organs.

Pranayama helps to increase the rate of removal of waste from the body and, hence, protecting the body from the impact of toxic substances. If the toxic substances that are supposed to be thrown out during exhalation are not thrown out, they get into the bloodstream again. This happens especially when we do shallow breathing because we don't exhale completely, leaving toxic substances inside the lungs. Proper exhalation is more important than inhalation. The human body can inhale easily; the real trick is emptying the lungs through exhalation because it has the waste products in it.

Pranayama gives great focus on exhalation. Pranayama boosts the circulation of blood throughout the body and takes away a big workload from the heart. Proper circulation of blood throughout the body helps blood to carry oxygen and nutrients to all parts of the body, nourishing them and helping to keep them healthy.

Eight qualities of breathing:

1. Silent—no noise while breathing.
2. Fine—no huffing and puffing.
3. Slow—one can feel the inhalation retention and exhalation clearly.
4. Deep—diaphragm moves up and down as a result of deep breaths.
5. Long—long enough to get the feeling as though the lungs are getting full during inhalation and empty after exhalation.
6. Soft—no tension in the nose and throat.

7. Continuous—no pauses.
8. Even—equal time for inhalation and exhalation.

There are many ways to exercise control over your breath. One of them is walking breath. This is a wonderful yoga practice that can be done right in the middle of daily life, and *integrates* body, breath and mind.

You count internally the number of steps you take while inhaling and exhaling, and align this with the steps you are taking while walking.

This activity can be used as a training game as well. The steps are as follows:

1. Ask all participants to walk in a circle. Suddenly, ask them to stop wherever they are. Repeat this a couple of times.
2. Ask the participants to walk randomly. This time ask them to walk one step per breath. Do this for 30 seconds.
3. While the participants are walking randomly, ask them to walk two steps per breath. Do this for 30 seconds.
4. While the participants are walking randomly, ask them to walk three steps per breath. Do this for 30 seconds.
5. While the participants are walking randomly, ask them to walk four steps per breath. Do this for 30 seconds.
6. While participants are walking randomly, ask them to walk five steps per breath. Do this for 30 seconds.
7. While participants are walking randomly, ask them to walk six steps per breath. Do this for 30 seconds.
8. Reverse the sequence.

At the end of this activity, you will understand the integration of body, mind and breath.

What is common among all great thinkers?

It is a form of awareness that gave rise to Archimedes' eureka moment, Isaac Newton's insights into gravity, Einstein's theory of relativity, and humanity's great businesses, such as Amazon by Jeff Bezos. A mind free from chaotic thoughts is all that you need to be in line with Archimedes, Newton or Einstein. Their inventions were not accidents; they were the results of relaxed minds under a tree or in a bath tub. Awareness and mindfulness come through a relaxed mind.

"Mindfulness liberates more time than it consumes."

Many times, we struggle to control new thoughts. To control your thoughts, first you need to create space in your mind. If you tried meditation, did your mind become calm during meditation or was it like a butterfly flitting from one place to another? Almost everyone's mind becomes chaotic during their initial attempts at meditation. This reveals the mind's inner turmoil and innate desire to think at a faster rate. Sit quietly for a moment and see if there is any space for new thoughts. Your mind is designed to think. That's what it does. It's not surprising that it doesn't calm down easily. During meditation, slowly and gently thoughts start crystallising.

Breath plays a vital role in creating a chaotic mind. Restricting the breath causes the body to tense up, and the mind senses this and becomes increasingly wary and stressed. This then restricts the breath, which becomes faster and shallower. So even the slightest restriction to free-flowing breath can feedback into the deepest reaches of the mind to create some low level of stress and anxiety, which prevents the mind from relaxing.

Alternate nostril breathing and left/right brain thinking

When we inhale, inhaling through each nostril influences the two halves of the brain. Inhaling through the left nostril influences right brain activities, and inhaling through the right nostril influences left brain activities.

Left nostril/right brain activities	Right nostril/left brain activities
Associative thinking	Mathematical reasoning
Creative, calm, silent work	Physical activities
Drinking water	Eating
Leaving home	Returning home
Rearranging furniture	Doing accounts
Working with shapes or forms	Working with words and numbers
Nonverbal communication	Speaking, debating
Singing, playing, composing or listening to music	Reading, writing, studying or listening to words

Unfortunately, when breathing is in auto-mode, either we take shallow breaths or one of the nostrils is blocked, which impacts the functioning of the respective half of the brain.

The body, breath and mind are linked. So if there are irregularities in the breath, such as jerks, pauses, shallowness and noisiness in the breath, they are being caused by the mind. The mind can go in many directions within split seconds, which causes irregularities in the breath. The breath and body simply cannot operate without receiving instructions from the mind. So, if the breath is irregular, it is because of the irregularities in the mind.

Working with breath helps the mind: The beautiful thing is that if you eliminate the irregularities from the physical breath, it has an extremely beneficial effect on the mind as well. When the breath becomes smooth, continuous (without pauses), slow and quiet, the mind comes along, and also becomes calm and peaceful. The body also comes along and relaxes much more easily.

Breathing correctly at work helps to improve productivity, creativity, our decision-making capability and prevents fatigue.

Pratyahara—sensory control and withdrawal

Our five senses act as extended arms of the mind. These senses receive the information and pass it on to the mind, and then the mind reacts accordingly. Without the mind, our senses do not have any existence. Imagine if there was no mind. Our eyes would get no meaning from whatever they see. They would become a useless organ. Some people have a habit of sleeping with their eyes open. For them, even if their eyes are open their mind doesn't receive any input. So the human body has the capability of detaching the mind from our senses, even though it is not easy. Similarly, it is possible to detach the mind from our senses when our senses do not react to the mind.

Sensory control means not letting our senses react to the thoughts in the mind. It does not mean suppressing the senses but culturing and civilising them. This plays an important role to achieve concentration. Sensory withdrawal means withdrawal of senses from their external objects. In this state, information perceived through our senses does not distract the mind.

Dharana—concentration

Concentration is holding the mind on something, either inside the body or outside the body. When the mind succeeds on focusing on one thing, without letting other things enter our mind, that becomes concentration. For example, when you hear the bird sounds among all the other sounds around you, and try to listen only to that sound, and you succeed even though that sound may not be the loudest, that is concentration. In concentration, the mind just focuses on one thing. The mind discriminates one object from others. This capability of discrimination is concentration.

Yama, niyama, pranayama and asana are the external parts of concentration, meditation and blissful absorption. These four practices (yama, niyama, pranayama and asana) bring necessary fitness and capability to achieve concentration.

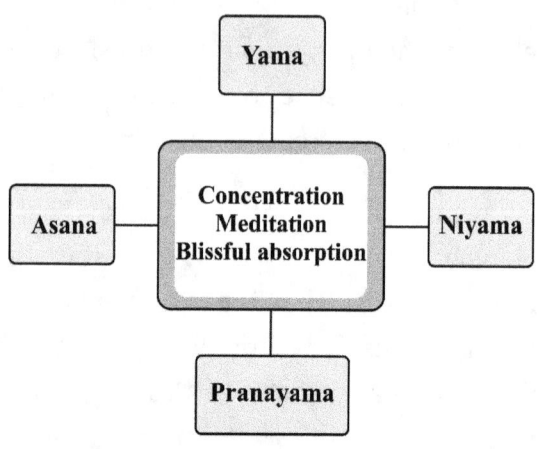

Fig- Internal vs external aspects of yoga

Let's play a game to understand concentration. You can play this game with your family members or team members as part of a team-building exercise.

Ask participants to walk randomly in the room and follow your instructions.

1. First round:
   - Ask them to stop. Again instruct them to walk for a few seconds.
   - Repeat it a couple of times.

- Now change the instruction. Ask them to walk when you say stop, and stop when you say walk. Do this for a minute.
2. Second round:
   - Now introduce new activities—clapping and jumping.
   - Ask them to clap when you say clap, and ask them to jump when you say jump.
   - Now change the instruction. Ask them to jump when you say clap and clap when you say jump.
3. Third round:
   - Ask them to walk when you say walk, and stop when you say stop.
   - Ask them to clap when you say clap, and ask them to jump when you say jump.

All you need is twelve seconds

I usually go for lunch in a park close to my office. Most of the time I see a gentleman meditating in the park. I was curious as to how he can meditate during lunch hour and wanted to know more about him. One day I went to speak to him immediately after he finished his meditation. He told me how he manages it.

He follows a twelve-seconds rule. This is probably the easiest way to understand and start practising meditation. All you need to do is fix your mind at the centre for twelve seconds. That's it. That is the first step towards meditation.

The process is like this:

1. Fix your mind for twelve seconds at the centre. That will be one cycle of concentration.
2. Twelve such cycles of concentration will be one cycle of meditation.
3. Twelve cycles of meditation will be blissful absorption (highest state of meditation).

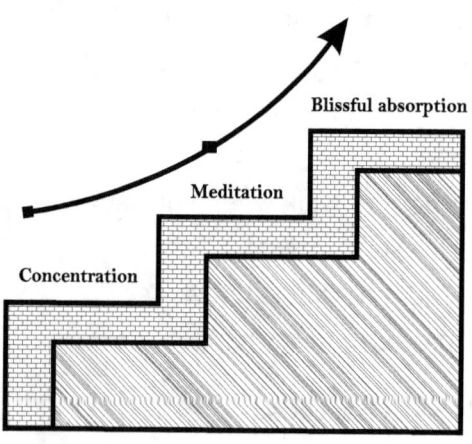

Fig.- Steps in meditation

When the concentration is sustained, it becomes meditation. In meditation, peace and relaxation are experienced. When meditation is sustained, the peaceful mind experiences detachment from joys and sorrows and gets into total absorption, and that is blissful absorption. Blissful absorption is the ultimate state of yoga.

Dhyana—meditation

"Dhyanenatmani pashyanti"

Through meditation self is seen.

—Bhagavad Gita

Power of emptiness:

Meditation is all about making your mind still. A still mind becomes a fertile ground for new thoughts.

A still mind is like zero. When it's just zero it's nothing. Zero is emptiness. Use the same zero next to a number and you will understand the power of zero. Similarly, an empty mind is nothing, but when you join this empty mind to positive thoughts, you will see the power of emptiness.

You will often observe that writers, poets and music composers always disconnect themselves from the rest of the world to focus on their work. In school and university we also use quiet libraries to focus on our studies. But when we get into the corporate world we forget the simple power of quietness. Quietness means there are no distractions, so the mind can focus on what you want to do.

When Archimedes was alone and quiet, that's when the idea of Archimedes' principle came to his mind. When Newton was sitting alone under the apple tree, that's when he came up with the idea of gravitational force. You would experience similar eureka moments in your life when you have fewer distractions.

They say that you should keep a pen and paper next to your bed as you might get ideas when you are resting. When we're in bed our mind and body are relaxed and that's why we tend to get ideas.

Zen gardens and room décor in Japan are designed to still and empty the mind, by relaxing the mind and allowing emptiness to rise naturally in the mind. We don't have to find a Zen garden, go in a bathtub naked, sit under an apple tree or lie in bed to relax the mind. A simple meditation will have a similar or better effect.

The mind is like the sky. A rainbow could be seen in the sky. Clouds will come and go but it doesn't affect the sky. Clouds could be dark, white and full of water or hold less water. Clouds can form different shapes. When the sky is covered by clouds that's when it starts raining. You can't see the blue sky if the sky is covered with clouds. Those clouds can cause thunderstorms, and cloudbursts can cause havoc on land. When clouds collide, the collision may create lightning. The sky can look like a big blue umbrella without any cloud. At night it is full of blinking stars. But the sky remains the sky. Things change but it doesn't affect the sky.

Thoughts are like clouds. Thoughts come and go. Good thoughts, bad thoughts, all types of thoughts. Let these thoughts come and go, don't hold onto them. If you hold onto thoughts it can cause a disturbance. The severity of the disturbance caused by these thoughts depends on how long you hold onto the thoughts for. The mind can become stormy, it can become calm. The mind can be flooded with thoughts, or it could be without any thoughts. The key is to not hold onto the clouds called thoughts.

I have heard many people say that they can't meditate. They can't stop thoughts coming into their mind. You can't stop clouds coming over the sky. It's a natural phenomenon. Similarly, thoughts will not stop coming. The key is to not pay attention to them so that they will vanish. When you empty a glass full of water, you still see some droplets of water in the glass. Similarly, when you meditate, you may still have some tiny thoughts somewhere in the mind. But the very fact that a huge chunk of mind will be empty, that is the biggest achievement.

One of the important principles of innovation, as suggested by Steve Jobs, is connecting the dots. That is, bringing different ideas together. Our mind is full of information. When we meditate we are looking deep inside the mind. They say that through meditation, self is seen. During meditation, lots of information may surface in terms of memory. When random information from some corners of the mind surfaces, it may join with some other piece of information, which may give rise to new ideas. That's why when we are stressed, we can't come up with the ideas, but when we are relaxed we come up with lots and lots of ideas that we can't keep track of. Just like a warehouse manager can recall the location of various parts in a huge warehouse based on his experience of visiting it many times and gathering the information during every visit, similarly every time we meditate we go to the deepest level of our mind, where all the information is stored, and thus don't lose track of any information stored in the warehouse of our mind. A regular visit to this deepest level through meditation helps to retrieve information whenever needed.

I was working for a consulting firm and we had to submit a proposal to a big bank. My boss arranged a conference call to brainstorm ideas. There were four people on the call: my boss from the United States, one person from India, one person from London and myself in Australia. My boss gave us a brief about the project and then gave us two minutes to come up with ideas. That was the weirdest situation in my life because I was on the train. No one came up with any ideas in those two minutes. Finally, we all agreed to spend a few hours coming up with ideas. This is a typical scenario in the corporate world. You can't expect people to come up with creative ideas by pressurising them. It is important that they have enough space in their mind to come up with creative ideas.

There was a gardener who was giving a gardening lesson to some kids. The first lesson he taught was how to remove weeds from the garden and then plant the seeds. "If you don't weed the land, it may destroy the seeds," he said. "Similarly, when the plants grow, you need to remove weeds regularly as they will keep popping up. You have to put in effort to plant the trees that you want, but weeds will grow automatically. To keep the garden beautiful, you need to keep removing weeds every now and then." Your mind is like a garden and your thoughts are plants and weeds. Good thoughts are like plants, and negative thoughts are like weeds. To maintain the growth of positive thoughts, every now and then you need to keep removing negative thoughts.

Benefits of meditation:

- To remain calm and clear-sighted under pressure.
- To enhance creativity.
- To enhance mental focus.
- To make better decisions.
- To sleep better.
- To renew the courage necessary to follow your path through life.
- To enhance mental and physical resilience.
- To cope with the angst of making an important decision.
- To ward off or relieve anxiety, stress and unhappiness.
- To live a good life that is meaningful and broadly happy.

Beautiful thoughts are like flowers. You need to arrange them properly to make a more beautiful picture out of them. So it's a ritual. Meditation is a ritual for arranging beautiful thoughts together.

"When it's stormy outside, stay inside. If things outside are not good, meditate."

One-pointed concentration

If you are playing and get bruised, sometimes you may not realise it until you see the bruise or someone tells you about it. That is because of your concentration on the game. On the contrary, when a doctor tells you a syringe is about to be injected into your body, you feel every movement of it as you concentrate on the injection. For example, some people feel the pain even before the syringe touches their body; they create that experience in their mind.

When you are watching an interesting movie, you may not be able to listen if somebody is calling you; you may not be able to smell if something is burning in the kitchen; you may not be able to sense if a mosquito is biting you. All these are examples of one-pointed concentration. Similarly, sometimes when you're driving, you may not be able to observe if someone is honking at you, or waving at you; that's what happens when we don't concentrate on driving, which can lead to fatal accidents. All these examples prove that there is a time when our senses become detached from our mind. When you are meditating the goal is to detach the mind from those senses so that they don't distract you. One-pointed concentration is about bringing all of your attention and focus to one point/thing.

When you feel lonely and miserable, if you read a good, interesting and absorbing book, or watch a TV show or paint, sing or dance, your concentration brings about the steadiness of mind that relieves you from the distress of your feelings and helps the healing process. So anything that facilitates concentration, reflection and inward absorption is going to heal the problems of a disturbed and imbalanced self.

We carry so many toxins in our memories; feelings we have stored away and allowed to stagnate and fester. We get used to carrying this sack of rubbish around, and we even conclude that it's just part and parcel of our character.

When you empty the mind, you also empty the toxins of memory.

Is meditation possible?

A car can be unlocked with a remote key. The moment you press the button, the car is unlocked. But if the battery in the remote is out then even if you have the remote, and you keep pressing the button, the car will not be unlocked. The battery in the remote plays an important role in passing the signal from the remote to the car. A battery can connect the remote to the car as well as disconnect with its power.

The body has various sense organs. When an eye sees something, that image is passed on to the brain and we see that

135

thing. Our brain can see only when the image captured by the eyes is passed on to the brain. Many people sleep with their eyes open. Yet they don't see anything, even if the eyes capture an image, because in that state the brain does not sense the image. Sometimes when we are lost in thought, we keep looking at something, but we don't notice anything about it. Even if our eyes capture something, it doesn't reach the brain. Similarly, we may play songs at a loud volume, but still we may not listen to the songs if the sound is not passed on to the brain.

We have an inherent capacity to disconnect our brain from the senses of sensory organs just like the remote of a car. We can switch it on and off depending on our will. And we do it many times during the day without even realising it. The phrase "selective hearing" also denotes the same thing.

So it is definitely possible to disconnect our sensory organs from our mind. When we can disconnect our senses, we will be in a meditative state.

When I was a kid I was always fascinated by the illusion of a moving train created on a stationary train. Watching a moving train from a stationary train always gave the feeling as if the other train was stationary and the one I was in was moving. The illusion stayed until I looked on the opposite side of my train. Thoughts are like that moving train, while our body is like a stationary train. That moving train may speed up, slow down, make a sound or create many effects that will make us feel that

that's happening to our train. We will understand reality only after looking away from the moving train. Similarly, moving thoughts make us feel the same effect on our body. Just as by looking away from the moving train we notice that we are still stationary, moving away from the moving thoughts will help us bring us into the present situation or mindfulness. It's just that we need to realise the difference between a moving train and a stationary train.

How do we meditate?

While there are different ways to meditate, for most people meditation is all about not allowing any thoughts to take over the mind. That can happen only when you reach an advanced state. But you can still train the mind to avoid thoughts. As you empty the water from the glass it still has some drops in the bottom. Similarly, even if you empty your mind it will still have some thoughts. But over time they will reduce.

Some of the ways to meditate:

1. Abhyasa and vairagya—regular practice and renunciation: when you meditate for two minutes, for those two minutes you have to tell your mind just to concentrate on your breath and forget about the rest of the world. Practise this regularly and those two minutes will start increasing in time.
2. Yoga—try to balance your body in various yoga postures.

3. Pranayama—it automatically takes you to a meditative state.

4. Mental tiredness—if you practise the above areas, you will also experience a point when the mind gets tired of thinking about all the thoughts entering it. Let it be. That means the more you meditate, the more chances the mind will have to stop thinking. Just like when we are in bed, we will think, but eventually we will sleep. Similarly, the mind will eventually slow down with thinking.

Western superstition

I was attending a vegan festival with my Western friends. It was interesting to learn about the vegan perspective. The festival was all about the benefits and ways of living a vegan lifestyle. There was a tremendous amount for me to learn. I learned a lot about nature and my own body, too.

One night, when it was almost midnight, one of my friends asked me if I would like to join in some midnight meditation. I had heard of full-moon meditation but midnight meditation was a new term for me, and I was keen to know more about it. I joined the group. We all walked up the hill towards a cave-like structure. As the festival was away from the city and in a remote area, there was absolute silence. We were walking in the moonlight. That itself was so amazing.

We reached the cave-like structure and sat in a circle. I was excited to learn a new way of meditation. While we were quiet, one person rolled some weed and lit it and started passing it among the circle. That was a shock for me. I skipped it as I'd never tried it before and had no intention of smoking weed to meditate. After a couple of rounds of smoke, soft music was started and we all closed our eyes and followed the guided meditation. I felt like asking the question, if you need to alter your state of mind through an external substance to meditate, then how can it be meditation?

There was one more incident at my friend's place. I was visiting him and we didn't have any plans over that weekend, so he suggested we meditate. I was happy to do so. Then I saw two glasses of wine. We drank and tried to meditate. I could not.

This is what I call Western superstition: the belief that weed, alcohol and drugs are a means to achieve a meditative state. None of the original texts about mediation prescribe any mind-altering substances. I also heard the justification from some that yogis in the Himalayas use weed to meditate, so it's okay to smoke weed for meditation, but I personally feel it's just a lame excuse. Also, many people fail to understand that not everyone who stays in the Himalayas, has dreadlocks and claims to be a yogi, is actually a yogi! So you need to be careful who you follow for your yogic journey. If weed helped in meditation, all yoga gurus would have prescribed it.

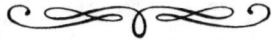

Chapter 3

A yogic lifestyle

"The knowledge of self is the only way to liberation."

One of the major categories of disease that we all suffer from is called lifestyle disease. Our current lifestyle is causing this disease. This lifestyle includes physical inactivity and eating habits that have a direct impact on our physical and mental health. Electronic gadgets only aggravate the problem. Many studies have proven the impact of mobiles on kids' growth and minds. While we leverage the technology, we need to make sure that we don't become slaves to it. That's where a yogic lifestyle comes into the picture. A yogic lifestyle does not mean living a primitive life in a hermitage; it means doing everything that is good for your body and mind.

Just like a caterpillar covers itself with silk created by its own mouth, human beings wrap themselves with the stress created by their own minds. Caterpillars become butterflies with their own desire by breaking the silk; similarly, we can liberate ourselves by our own desire by breaking the bonds of stress created by us wrapped around ourselves.

140

The human body can be divided into the following systems:

- Respiratory
- Circulatory
- Digestive
- Hormonal
- Reproductive
- Excretory

Good health comes from the proper functioning of all of these systems and related organs. Yogic practices help to maintain the proper functioning of these systems through various methods. They also maintain good communication between body and mind, which is essential for peace and happiness.

The treasure

Mind, body and breath are the most precious assets of human life and they should therefore be treated quite literally as genuine treasures—conserved, protected, loved and valued. Most people take their bodies for granted and wear them out as engines of pleasure, rather than taking loving care of them. Yogic life gives the utmost importance to these treasures.

Life

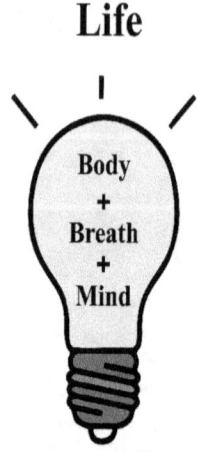

Fig.- Treasures of human life

The mind is the most mysterious thing. We all refer to it but no one knows where it is and what it looks like. There is no one definition of mind. Brain and heart are sometimes used as a substitute of mind, but they are not. Physicists also struggle to define the mind.

When I was in university, my friends and I used to write secret messages to each other, just for fun. There was nothing actually secret. We used to make the paper wet and then write on the paper with a pen without ink. The pressure created an impression on the paper, which couldn't be seen when the paper was dry. You could see the impressions only when the paper was wet.

Impressions on our mind are like those impressions on paper. They are there but you can't see them.

Describing the mind is difficult:

The mind is a crazy little thing that is very big.
It's here and the next moment it's there.
It is in your control but it is out of control.
It cannot be touched but it can be felt.
It can't be seen but it can be sensed.

Breath and food give us energy. Energy helps us live life. Yet millions of people can't live beyond thirty-five to forty years because of misuse of energy. It could be an overdose, accident because of speeding, death punishment because of crime or war, a contagious disease, etc. Their energy is misdirected through anger, hatred, jealousy and greed. All these acts are to fulfil small desires. The energy dissipates and will not be available to help them achieve joy. A yogic lifestyle focuses on the use of energy in the right direction and places. Yogic life is not using energy in the wrong way.

The aims of a yogic life:

- Doing your duty by living in the right way.
- Self-reliance—earning your own living.
- Pleasures of love and human enjoyment.
- Freedom.
- Detachment—the practice of detachment means detaching from the sufferings of everyday life. Detach from your office role as soon as you reach home and you will forget all the stress accumulated during the day at work.

Certain qualities, known as healthy and healing qualities of consciousness, nurture the mind, they are:

1. Maitri—Friendliness
2. Karuna—Compassion
3. Mudita—Joy
4. Upeksa—Indifference or neutrality

Consciousness vs partial consciousness

Consciousness has many definitions and is still difficult to understand. The most important goal of yogic life is to achieve consciousness. The simplest definition of consciousness could be:

"When you become sensitive towards everything around you, you achieve consciousness."

There is consciousness and there is unconsciousness. We spend our life in between these two stages being partially conscious.

We are conscious when we decide to be conscious of everything, such as what we eat, what we do, what we speak. Most of the time in our day-to-day life, we are not conscious about what we do, but we know what we are doing. That is what I call partial consciousness. When we become sensitive to everything around us, our every action will be thoughtful action.

We partially live in the past, partially in the present and partially in the future, which leads to partial consciousness. What is the past? Memories. What is the future? Imagination. Our life is squashed between the past and future so we lose the ability to use the direct perception of what really is now, the present.

Where do we go wrong? Consciousness has three functions:

1. Perception—how we perceive, know and recognise.
2. Decision—impulse to initiate action.
3. Action—what and how we act.

Yoga is the process of creating awareness about perception, decision and action by stilling the movement and fluctuations of the mind that disturb our consciousness. It's like when our house is gloomy because the windows are dirty. We don't say there is a problem with the sun, we clean the windows! Therefore, yoga cleanses the lens of perception. What lens we put on makes a difference to our decisions and actions. Ancient yogic literature talks about three nerves called sushumna, ida and pingala. These nerves are considered as the main channels of energy—keeping them unblocked helps to allow prana to move freely throughout the body. Yogic practices help to unblock these nerves. As per yogic literature, the sushumna nerve also helps to achieve consciousness.

"Madhya vikasat chidananda labhaha."

The unfolding of the central nerve (sushumna) gives rise to the bliss of consciousness.

This answers the question about what we do if we want to achieve consciousness.

Every person around you is significant

It was a good career move for me; I had become the head of a unit in a big organisation. My heart was full of pride. I felt great as I was at the right stage in my career at the right time. My manager was super nice, too. That was one reason I had joined the organisation. In the first week after joining, I was asked to familiarise myself with the office environment and settle down. After that week, my manager set up a quick catch-up to check how I was going. I prepared notes about many things—good things, bad things that needed improving, areas where my team could add more value, etc.—and I was ready to discuss everything in detail.

During the catch-up, surprisingly my manager wasn't keen to discuss my work and said, "I believe in your capabilities and I know you're doing well in terms of work, but I have a question: what is the name of our receptionist?" That was a tricky question, which I didn't expect. By now I knew almost everyone in my team. But I hadn't spoken to the receptionist after collecting my office pass on day one, even though I crossed reception every day. That was the day I leaned my biggest leadership lesson: *everyone around you is significant*. As a leader you need to give importance to everyone around you. Everyone plays a significant role in your achievement, some directly, others indirectly. Be friendly to everyone in the organisation. Everyone deserves your attention and care, even if all you do is just smile and say hello. This was the best advice I had received in my life.

It may sound like the advice of a professor to his/her students studying a management course, but look around and we will understand why many people still need to be told the importance of this behaviour. For a yogi, everyone is equally important, irrespective of designation, age, etc.

Goodness is in our cells

The human body is made up of millions and millions of cells. There are more than 200 different types of cells. Millions of cells die every minute and millions of new cells are born at the same time. All these cells do their work diligently. White blood cells are an important part of the body. Their volume is roughly 7,000 white blood cells per microlitre of blood. The function of white blood cells is to protect the body against both infectious disease and foreign invaders. A white cell can distinguish between invading enemy bacteria and harmless pollen. White cells protect the body. These cells ensure the welfare of the body and, when required, offer to die fighting foreign invaders. Similarly, different cells from different organs of the body, such as the lungs, liver, kidneys and brain, perform their actions and keep us alive by risking their own survival. All cells recognise the importance of each other and help each other to perform their functions. Every cell acts to keep the body; that is, the rest of the cells, alive, and that's the nature of every cell in the body—to help other cells. They do everything to help other cells live. Our body is made up of cells, and it means helping others is in our cells, it is in our nature. If cells become cancerous, this causes disease in the body. Similarly, if we harm others, we call it a mental disease. Yogic life is aligning yourself to the nature of your cells by helping others to live, and loving them.

Who is rich?

I took a small break from work once when I wanted to explore southern India as I had heard a lot about it. I decided to start from Bangalore, which is also known as the Silicon Valley of India.

One of my friends from my university days lives in Bangalore. We hadn't met for almost ten years as we were both busy building our corporate careers. When he understood that I was planning to visit Bangalore, he invited me to his house. When we were together in university we'd had so much fun, so I couldn't resist his offer.

I landed in Bangalore in the evening. I felt excited to see my friend after such a long time. My cab stopped in front of his house, well, it was like a bungalow, and that also in a city like Bangalore where people struggle to buy an apartment. I was happy to realise that he was doing well. As soon as I got out of my car, we both literally started jumping with joy. What a pleasure to meet a friend from my university days. I knew that he had a son, but as soon as I entered his house, a cute baby girl toddled towards me and extended her hand, asking for my hand. I presumed she wanted to show me something. My friend, his son, his wife and this baby girl, everyone was so excited to see me and wanted to grab a share of my attention. I felt like a superstar. My friend whispered in my ear, "I have adopted this baby." I looked at his face and I felt a sudden silence around me. I became quiet and lost for words. My friend whispered, "I will tell you the story later." I came down to my knees, held the shoulders of the little girl with both hands, and just hugged her. My eyes became teary. I didn't understand what was happening with my emotions. That little girl had been an orphan.

After dinner, my friend told me that after their first child, he and his wife had decided to adopt a baby girl. They didn't have any medical issues but it was their conscious decision to do something good for someone. They went against their family, friends and society and adopted this baby. She had been left at a remote railway station by her biological parents when she was just six months old. Some stranger gave her to the police and the police then handed her over to the nearest orphanage. This process took four to five days. A six-month-old baby, without a mother, in the hands of a stranger for four to five days and then in an orphanage. I felt the cruelty of the world and some sensation of anger against someone somewhere inside of me.

My friend met her when she was eight to nine months old. When they saw her for the first time, she just leapt into my friend's arms as though she were saying please take me from here, I need love, I need parents... For my friend that was the best moment of his life to experience that unconditional and real love from an innocent child. At that moment they decided to adopt the girl.

Now she is so happy in her new family. That baby has a home, family and a future.

When two friends meet, most of the time they compare wealth, salary, organisation, title, cars, etc. Yet no matter how much money my friend earns, he is the richest among all of my friends, and no one can match the richness of his heart. He is the biggest example of compassion I have seen in my life.

A new business model—organisation without customers

Once a friend suggested visiting a restaurant called "Lentil as Anything" in Newtown, Sydney. Newtown is very close to Sydney's CBD, so my first impression of the restaurant was that it must be expensive.

We reached the restaurant and I was amazed to see the crowd. We had to wait for some time as the restaurant was full. But I liked the ambience. It was full of noise with music in the background, but the noise was pleasant. The noise was similar to that of a college canteen. The place was full of energy, and there was one unique thing—most of the faces were happy.

It was our turn. We were guided to a table and then given the menu. To my surprise, the menu was without any prices. Maybe my friend realised what I was thinking.

He said, "You pay as you feel suitable for the food you have."
I was like, "What? Does that mean I can pay $1?"
The answer was, "Yes."
"And what if the customer doesn't pay?"
"No worries, it's up to you how much you want to pay."

I thought it must be funded by someone rich, but then I found out that "Lentil as Anything" is a not-for-profit community organisation. It's more than thirteen years old. It has five restaurants and is expanding. You can have breakfast, lunch and dinner there. It only has partners and no customers. Partners are:

- those who eat in the restaurant and give what they feel the food is worth
- those who donate
- volunteers.

It was such a wonderful place where artists could organise an exhibition, a creative person could showcase their talent, a student from hospitality could get experience and a hungry person could quench their hunger.

It is a unique financial model that is centred on the values of trust, generosity and respect, and which gives people the opportunity to eat out and be social regardless of their financial situation.

I saw people from all strata of society in the restaurant; homeless, backpackers, artists, office-goers, rich. I felt that there was respect for everyone, and that is what I would call compassion.

Fun—the missing element

Have you ever tried cappuccino with salt? I asked the participants in an innovation workshop I was holding.

Everyone gave me a weird look. I told them, "I did!" I then narrated the incident of how I mixed salt into a cappuccino and finished the cup. There was laughter in the room and it created the perfect grounds for me to continue my workshop and hook the audience with a smile for the rest of the day.

A couple of years back, I attended a town hall meeting by a CEO. The first slide of the presentation was about injuries, which he'd got while playing baseball. He went on to explain how his family members made fun out of these incidents. That created laughter and made everyone in the room comfortable and relaxed. The presentation went on for an hour and the CEO ended with a few more funny incidents from the cricket world. Every employee had a smile on their face at the end of the session.

At the start of my career, during training sessions, I tried to explain difficult concepts in the best possible way. Soon I realised, however, that you can bring life to the difficult concepts only with fun and humour.

"The fish" philosophy is based on a fun environment at the workplace. Many organisations create a fun environment by playing songs, making employees dance or whatever. Organisations like Google are famous for their workplace design.

Fun is the ace card. No one wants to be sad, lonely in their life. This is the basis for social networking sites like Facebook or Meetup. Apps with games are a "must have" on everyone's mobile. Still, the fun is missing at many places.

Somehow, many in the corporate world believe that not bringing a smile to their face or looking aggressive makes you more corporate, professional. Really?

Yogic life is all about achieving joy.

The absence of fun and too much routine are the root causes of stress. Routine can lead to boredom and boredom can lead to frustration. Frustration can lead to stress. While many organisations include programs to break the routines, this seems to be a once-in-a-while activity.

Yogic life believes in celebration; celebration of everything, every day. For example, the change of the season, the beginning/closure of events, such as geographical events like an eclipse. Every celebration is different. Some celebrations involve food, some involve fasting. Some celebrations involve respecting relationships, while others involve respecting nature. That's why life itself becomes a celebration. The corporate world has borrowed some of these concepts in the form of the celebration of a project start/end, a culture day, birthday celebrations, annual day, etc., but, still, this doesn't seem to be adequate for employees. It's high time we made every day a celebration while keeping the focus on productivity and efficiency.

Service others to find joy

Everyone has a side of sympathy and kindness. It's just that people flip between the sides and it depends on many circumstances.

A HR manager from one of the Fortune-500 organisations went to visit a monk. She was a little disturbed. She couldn't sleep properly at night and mentioned this situation to the monk. She was responsible for the HR of an organisation that had grown so rapidly they'd had to hire many people urgently. She had come up with a referral scheme, called "Each one brings ten", in which existing employees attracted talent to the organisation from their network and in turn they would get a handsome referral commission. The company had bright prospects so existing employees convinced many bright candidates in their network to join them. Things worked. Soon the organisation became a Fortune-500 organisation. People took pride in associating themselves to the brand.

However, things turned ugly after some time. A change in technology and competition affected the rapid growth of the organisation and its profits started declining at a rapid pace. To manage the losses, HR had to make people redundant. That same year the recession hit the world. Those people who were the best talent in the market suddenly realised they had no place in the market. They found it difficult to get a job. Two redundant employees committed suicide as they could not cope with the financial pressure and the social taboo of being unemployed. Many other redundant employees went through more or less similar bad phases of their life. The HR manager felt she was responsible for their plight. The picture of family members of the people who'd committed suicide made her restless and she couldn't get proper sleep. She felt that somehow her HR strategy went wrong and she was responsible for the redundancies.

Guilt and punishment are linked in our society. If you are guilty, you get punished. This woman felt guilty but there was no punishment for her as she'd followed the rules. So in the court of law she was not guilty, but she was guilty in her own eyes. Whomever she spoke to—colleagues, family members—all tried to tell her that she wasn't guilty and she should forget it, but it didn't help.

When the monk heard the story, he said, "I agree that you are guilty." The HR manager was shocked. The monk said exactly what she wanted to hear; she was guilty. And she should get punished to get out of this guilt. The punishment was to offer service to others in all possible way, irrespective of age, gender, race, etc. Service could be chatting with aged people in a care home or offering foster care, or just helping random people who were in need.

The HR manager started helping people. Every time she helped someone, their reaction helped her to feel the joy inside her. She started finding joy in small acts, like giving a hand to an elderly person to push their shopping cart while they were crossing traffic lights, or buying lunch for a homeless person and just spending a couple of minutes chatting with them, etc. She never looked back.

I remember my first visit to Australia. My friend was supposed to pick me up at the airport but something urgent had come up and he asked me to reach his home on my own. I just had the bus number and the final address with me. I had to change the bus in the centre of the city. I came out of the airport and struggled to reach the right bus stand. Finally, I located the stand and the bus was there. I quickly boarded with my two big and one small bags. I asked the driver if it would go into the city, just to make sure. After confirming, he asked me for three dollars. I took out a 100-dollar bill (after all, that's how you get money when you're travelling overseas). The driver apologised saying he didn't have change. But he pointed me to a ticket vending machine near the stand and suggested getting a ticket from the machine. I got off the bus, tried inserting the 100-dollar bill, but the machine could only accept a maximum of a 20-dollar bill. I was lost and didn't know what to do.

There were two teenagers nearby. I approached them for change, and even they didn't have any. Frustration and confusion were obvious on my face. There was an elderly man who asked what I was struggling for. I told him about the trouble. He pulled a 5-dollar bill from his pocket and handed it over to me. I pushed the 100-dollar bill towards him but he lovingly said, "That's okay." I didn't feel good accepting money but I had no choice. I insisted he take the 100-dollar bill, but he refused. He said, "Son, it looks like you're new here. Enjoy your stay." That really touched my heart. I thanked him and boarded the bus and got my ticket.

I got off the bus in the centre of the city and the first thing I did was go into a supermarket to get change. I got two 50-dollar bills. So at least then I thought I wouldn't have a problem. I boarded another bus and, to my disappointment, the driver didn't have enough change. But he asked me to take a seat. A passenger on the bus gave me the change. While getting down at my stop, I told the driver that I hadn't paid, but he said, "That's okay." He also helped me to get the luggage off the bus as he realised I was struggling to manage everything.

I got off the bus and there was literally no one around. I had the address but didn't know where to go as my mobile didn't have a local SIM to access the internet. I saw an old lady coming towards me. When I said hi, she said she was about to ask if I needed any help as I looked puzzled. I showed her the address and asked for directions. She asked me to follow her to her car and she got a map from her car. But she was struggling to locate the address. She asked me to wait for a minute as her husband would have a smartphone, which would be easier. Her husband arrived and upon looking at the address in the smartphone map, he said it was a couple of minutes away. He offered me a lift, even though I didn't want to bother them anymore. But he insisted. And I was at the doorstep of my friend's house with lots of gratitude for all the people I had met during my short trip.

Contact and connection and socialising

The advent of social media has changed our perception about connection. These days, connection is more about connecting through social media, even though you may never have met or interacted with that person in real life. That's why you get it as "request for connection".

Many times we feel a connection when we meet someone for the first time. Something leaves a deep impression on us and we feel connected to that stranger and we get along instantly. But this happens rarely as although we meet/see many strangers during the day, we hardly establish any lasting connections with these new faces. When we join a new organisation we are introduced to many people. The first couple of days you may see a smile from these new people. But soon you become part of the crowd and the smiles disappear and egos surface. This happens because of the absence of connection. Connection is all about dropping your ego and giving that smile.

Establish the connection, not the contact.

Living with nature

The life of a corporate person is controlled by the calendar. For example, the weekend is for relaxation, leave is to travel and spend time with family. A yogi, however, lives his/her life in alignment with nature's cycles. For example, mediating during a full moon is considered effective. Early morning and evenings have special importance and are treated as more beneficial. What and how much to eat depends on the time of day, etc. Pivotal periods of peak energy are the summer and winter solstices, which are the longest and shortest days of the year respectively, and spring and autumn equinoxes when the Earth's equator comes closest to the sun in its elliptical orbit length. These are excellent times to harvest energies. The eleventh day of a fortnight in the lunar month is considered to have importance in yogic life.

Just like the phase of the moon affects the tides in the ocean, it affects the atmospheric pressure as well. According to atmospheric scientists, air pressure rises to the extreme during a full moon and new moon because of the combination of the orbital path of the sun, moon and the Earth. Air pressure is the lowest on the eleventh day of every fortnight in a lunar month. To avoid the adverse impact of air pressure on the digestive system, yogis abstain from food on this day. This day is also considered a good time to exercise control over our sense organs. Abstinence from food gives an opportunity to exercise control over the tongue sense organ. Temporary abstinence from food also has the power to cleanse and heal the body.

Similarly, there are many events based on the lunar calendar. Many countries, such as India, China, Japan, Korea and Vietnam, use the lunar calendar to celebrate many festivals, including New Year.

Yogis start the day early. Most others do the exact opposite. Everything is suitable for night-time to give your body the proper rest it deserves. Staying awake until late and then getting up late disturbs the whole cycle and we go against nature. We force our body to follow what we want, not what it needs. A proper sleep plays an important part in maintaining the proper functioning of the body. Lack of proper sleep is the cause of many ailments. Time spent in bed without proper sleep is a waste of time.

Yogis believe in going to bed early and rising early. They want to meet the day as early as possible. They know that the morning time is the most productive time of the day. Be it for exercise, study, meditation, yoga or creative work.

The concept of daylight saving itself signifies the importance of every hour when we have sunlight. Yogis use the daylight saving concept throughout their life as they don't look at the clock but focus on getting up before the sun rises in the sky.

Certain locations on the planet are known as power spots, which can produce remarkably powerful effects on the human energy system when yogic habits are practised there, particularly when they are combined with special events in nature. Some mountains are more powerful than others due to their specific location relative to the sun, moon, planets, stars and various constellations. There is a high negative-ion count in the air, clarity of light and purity of water. The five sacred mountains of china—Omei shan, wu tai Shan, Tai shan, Hua shan and Chung Shan—Mount Shasta in California, Uluru in central Australia, Mount Ararat in Iraq, and many others, such as the Himalayas, are examples of mountains auspiciously located for internal energy work and advanced spiritual practice.

In ancient times, when there was a much better understanding of these aspects of locations, all-important edifices such as temples and palaces were built precisely on these locations as they were known to be power spots.

The first time I understood the true meaning of mindfulness

It was a Friday. Friday is a casual day in most organisations, and the same was the case in my organisation. Casual dress and Friday make the mood more casual.

A meeting request from our Function Head popped up on my laptop screen. It was an all-hands meeting. We'd already had one all-hands meeting just the previous week, so everyone raised their eyebrows in curiosity. Normally unplanned, all-hands meetings are a signal of organisational announcements. With not-so-great enthusiasm but out of curiosity, we joined the meeting.

The Function Head knew that we were all curious with the sudden meeting request, so straightaway he mentioned that there was a surprise.

"We are going to do an exercise," he told us in the meeting room.

We had already been chasing some milestones for the last few months and now he was talking of one more exercise. We forced a smile with some discomfort on our faces as if we were ready for additional work.

"So the exercise is like this. We will all go to the botanical gardens next to our office, take a walk around the garden and take photographs of anything we think is beautiful. If you think there is a tree or a flower that you feel is beautiful, try touching it and feel the texture and fragrance of that flower. Watch the leaves when they sway in the breeze. And share your experiences once you come back."

There was a big smile on our faces now. What kind of exercise is that? Something like we used to do in school. But the Function Head refused to reveal any further details. He also mentioned that we were free to go alone or buddy-up with a friend, or go as a team.

It was a winter's day and we had official permission to go to the botanical gardens. Whatever the objective of the exercise was, we were getting a break from work, so we were happy. We flocked to the coffee shop, picked up extra-hot coffees and headed to the botanical gardens. It was fun. We reached there in a group but then we naturally split up and went in different directions. I felt that a sense of competition and privacy led to the splitting of the group.

We walked around the gardens and took pictures. We often visited these gardens during our lunch breaks, but that day we observed everything. There were a few things that we must have subconsciously felt were beautiful on our previous walks, but we'd never paid much attention to them. That day we realised there were many things that were really beautiful and that we'd never noticed before.

We came back after an hour with great freshness and energy. The Function Head asked us to share our experiences. Almost everyone said the same thing: we never knew there are so many things that are so beautiful. Normally we just noticed the beautiful things that are really obvious, like bright flowers. But there are other beautiful things, too, such as carvings on the trunks of the trees, the way plants are planted, the combination of trees and plants, winding pathways and statues. At the end of the meeting, the Function Head smiled at all of us and said, "What you guys did today is called mindfulness. When we're busy or preoccupied with thoughts, we ignore many details.

What you did today was mindfulness by paying attention to many details. Now the next part of the exercise is to select any person at random—it has to be a random person from our office—and chat with him or her to understand how valuable that person's contribution is for the organisation."

Our jaws dropped. We soon realised that every day we speak to people with stereotypes in our mind based on our previous interactions, and sometimes that leads to problems. But this simple exercise was going to help us to change our perceptions.

Mindfulness will help you to think beyond stereotypes and understand your colleagues in a truer sense, to build the culture of collaboration. That is the real power of mindfulness at work.

Every small help matters

During one of my training sessions, there was this guy who was really attentive throughout the session. The training was on problem-solving techniques. It wasn't a really enjoyable session actually as it involved a lot of statistics.

This guy was trying to understand every concept in detail. I believed that you didn't really need to go into too many details in such training as long as you understood the application of the tools.

I caught up with him during the lunch break and asked him what made him go into such detail. Initially I thought perhaps it was to dominate office politics. With a smile he shook my hand and asked me to take the chair next to him.

"I need to tell you this," he said. "I was born in a country when it was going through war. We were three brothers living in a village that constantly saw bombing, gun battles and explosions. Since it was a tiny island country, we could not leave our village and go to some other place. We were a family of five: three kids and two parents. One day we kids woke up to a horrible scene in our courtyard. My parents were lying in a pool of blood. They were dead. While I was trying to understand what I was seeing, my eldest brother shouted at me and my sister to run from the scene. I don't know what he saw and why he asked this. We were so frightened that we all ran into the jungle without a second thought. We were in the jungle for almost a week. Only my elder brother knew where we were going. He used to disappear every day to meet someone. One night, he took us to a nearby beach where we all boarded a boat, along with at least 100 other people. We were leaving the country, for sure. We sailed for a couple days without food and water.

"We thought life was unfair to us. Then our boat hit a big storm. It overturned and everyone fell into the water. I don't remember what happened after that as I fell unconscious. When I opened my eyes I was in a hospital in a foreign country. I frantically searched for my brother and sister but couldn't find them. I was told that lots of people died in that accident.

"I grew up in that foreign land assuming my brother and sister were dead. There were many such family members separated from each other. There was a gentleman who created a directory of all people like me so that we could reconnect with our family members. I registered my details and forgot about it. Four or five years later, I went to refer to the directory and I got goosebumps when I saw the names of my brother and sister on the list. They were alive but in two different countries. Finally, we were reunited, thanks to the gentleman who took the effort to reunite families.

"So I try to proactively offer help whenever possible in all aspects of life because such proactive help by someone reunited me with my family. After this training I'm going to share my knowledge proactively with others in my organisation. Maybe it's not a big thing for me, but someone who receives that knowledge might be in need of it and will benefit from it. Who knows, someone may get promoted, or land a better job."

I was speechless and kept staring at his face. His eyes had that spark. I thought, *if everyone thinks like him, imagine how productive teams could be.*

Perfectionism is superficial

"If you want to do a really good thing, you have to make an effort to finish it and you will be close to perfect." - Unknown

When an artist is creating art, does perfection depend on the perception of the artist or others? Whether you try to prepare a document, create a new product or introduce a new service, you aim to perfect it. The definition of perfect is that you should be happy with your delivery, your manager should be happy, the head of department should be happy, the head of the organisation should be happy and the customer should be happy. So it's a long list of people who should be happy! What is perfect for one person may not be perfect for another, and that's what leads to stress and frustration.

There is a concept called interchangeability in mechanical engineering. It is used for manufacturing products at different locations and bringing them together at a third location to assemble and make into one product. The great challenge is that because two different parts are being manufactured in bulk quantity at two different locations, there could be a chance that they may not fit together well. In comes the concept of tolerance.

Tolerance is the specification given to a part to deviate from its original requirement. Tolerance is given because no part can be produced to exact requirements. Tolerance allows deviation and, as a result, better fitment with other products. Nothing in nature is absolutely perfect, so how can we expect to be perfect? We can strive for perfection but need not be obsessed with it. Obsession leads to stress. Give yourself some tolerance. Tolerance is such that even if you deviate from your target a little bit, you should still be happy with all the wholehearted effort you put in.

Sometimes you go into a meeting and present something and then feel stressed at the end as you think you might have missed something. But that's okay; you can't be perfect all the time because nothing is perfect.

"Your purpose is not to be perfect but to eliminate as many temptations and prejudices as possible."- Unknown

Breaking the boundaries of self-image

I went on a road trip with my childhood friend once, who is also a reputed doctor. We were camping during the trip. For my doctor friend it was a first-time experience; everything was new to him. He had to set up his own tent, make his own bed, cook his own food, etc. At the end of the trip he was tired from the physical exertion, but he was really happy. He came out of his doctor shoes for a few days and no one we met on the trip knew he was a doctor, and he also never introduced himself as a doctor. He finds it difficult to live such a life during his daily routine because he has to maintain his self-image as a doctor, and he has to live all the time in the boundaries of that image.

To feel good about yourself you need to renounce your self-image. When we are stuck in worrying about our self-image, which is created by ourselves, we look at everything from the lens of our self-image. This impacts our self-confidence.

When a woman flies a fighter jet we say she has high confidence, or she's brave. In reality, she just wants to fly fighter jets just like other pilots might. Self-confidence comes from renouncing your self-image as you purely focus on what needs to be done instead of focusing on what is right and what is wrong with respect to your own self-image. When a male actor performs the role of a female on the stage, we praise him for his confidence, but that confidence also comes from him renouncing his self-image during the act.

When you have to present in front of the senior leadership of your organisation, you might fumble, your hands might shake, your palms might get sweaty, you fidget... All this happens because you see the difference between the person next to you and yourself. These things don't happen when you are doing the same thing in front of your friends. You create your self-image as a junior in the organisation and that prevents you from being confident in front of your senior leadership.

The moment you renounce your self-image you will find yourself more open and relaxed. It's like asking an older person to join you to dance, and he/she joining without any hesitation because he/she renounces their self-image as "old" and, as a result, we feel they are more open.

One of the most important principles of yogic life is "Aham Brahmāsmi"; that is, "I am everything". Following this simple principle can change life drastically. When you are everything, you are nothing. When you think of you as only your body, then you will always be stuck with the pleasures and pains of your body. When you expand a little further and also think that you are also a father, mother, brother, sister, uncle to someone, etc., you gain another identity and you are stuck with the pains of pleasures of your relatives. Limiting your identity will limit your world to these people. When you keep expanding—a friend, a part of society, part of a country, part of the world—and take responsibility (care) for everything in the world, you will realise that your own pains and pleasures are trivial. When you reach that level, you become Mother Teresa, Baba Amte and Nelson Mandela. The whole world becomes your family.

When you find yourself responsible for everything around you, you will start caring for everyone and everything around you as your family. You will have compassion for animals, you will love plants and trees, and you will find yourself as an ocean of love.

Create a protective layer

A bushman in Australia was explaining the unique things about the bush to me. Among all the interesting things he mentioned, the most interesting thing that I picked up on is the behaviour of the trees.

The majority of Australia is prone to bushfires. Every year, hundreds of acres are destroyed in bushfires, but still you will find centuries-old trees in many areas. Trees have the unique ability to shed their skin ahead of summer. I first noticed it when the trunks of many trees had different colours; in between creamy white to reddish brown.

Just before the summer, trees shed the top layer of their skin. So if there is a fire, only the top layer gets burnt. The shed skin is fragile, but the new skin is tough. Another property is that the trunk with the new skin is very cold. I was told that if you are lost in the bush, you should hug the trunks to avoid dehydration, as hugging a cold trunk can help lower your body temperature.

Bushfires are a yearly phenomenon and the trees have adapted to this reality. We as human beings don't have the capability to shed our skin nor get burnt as we don't have to stay in one place. But, yes, every now and then circumstances create a fire of emotional imbalance and burn us from the inside. Just like the tree, if we do not create a self-protective mechanism, we will keep burning from within. Meditation and yoga make you strong internally, which help you to deal with the ups and downs of life. They create a protective layer around our mind, which won't let the fire of stress, anxiety and loss burn it.

Unfortunately, just like bushfires, we don't know when the tree will catch fire. Similarly, we can't predict when we will face fire, so we'd better be ready rather than getting destroyed by a sudden attack.

Shape employees' habits

Organisations are responsible for their employees' habits. For example, install a coffee machine and you will find someone who's never drank coffee before getting addicted to coffee. You will often hear people saying I got into this habit because my previous organisation had it. Similarly, when you provide facilities such as a gym or table tennis, you will find people use it, which is good for employees.

At the same time, the organisation is equally responsible for bad habits. Many times, goals are not clear, and that builds frustration. Constant restructuring and a high turnover of staff demotivates employees. Sometimes there are external factors that make organisations take these decisions, but gossip, politics and absenteeism continue the vicious cycle. This hampers both the organisation and individuals' productivity. The worst impact is on the mental health of the employees.

Change is constant, so helping employees cope with change is important. A negative mindset pollutes the environment. If thoughts are clouded, employees can't make proper decisions. This impacts the end customer.

There are often quiet rooms in organisations, where people can go to sit quietly for some time, take personal phone calls, just kill time, do a job search or stay away from everything and everyone.

Imagine having a dedicated meditation room where anyone can go, sit quietly for a few minutes, closing their eyes. The room could have a nice ambience with soft music, dim lighting, relaxing fragrances, etc. The room could be open to all, all the time, to meditate without disturbing others in the room.

Imagine the benefits of helping employees relax. They may:

- find answers to their problems
- come up with new ideas
- remember some important thing
- calm down
- feel happy.

All this will create an immense benefit for you and your organisation.

If an organisation can't help you with providing a meditation room, you can still try to find a quiet spot and meditate for yourself.

> "The existing level of thinking cannot solve the same level of problems else we would have had some part of the world absolutely stress free."

Minimalism

One of my friends was visiting me from Romania. He arrived with only one bag, whereas I carry at least two big bags each time I travel overseas. I was surprised by his small luggage. For his ten-day stay with me, he had everything he needed, even though it was just in one bag. He introduced me to the world of minimalism. Minimalism is living life with what you need and nothing in excess.

After understanding the definition of minimalism, I opened my cupboard and looked at my clothes. I had not worn some of them for almost a year or more, and still when I went out I couldn't stop the urge to buy new ones. My garage was full of stuff and so were the other parts of my house, with stuff I'd not used for months and years. That made me think, *Why am I sitting on so much stuff?*

The same thing happens to our minds as well. There is so much stuff that is not needed but still we collect it and keep it in our mind. Unwanted physical stuff can cause chaos in your house, while unwanted thoughts can cause chaos in your mind.

Look at your office drawers, files/pages on your desk, soft copies on your computer, and you will understand how we repeat the same thing in the office environment, too.

Five ways to do more with less

India's mission to Mars in 2014 was known for "Doing more for less". They say the cost of the Mars mission was equal to the cost of a Hollywood film. Doing more for less without compromising the end objective is also called frugal innovation.

Carlos Ghosn, Chairperson and CEO of the Renault–Nissan Alliance, coined the term "frugal engineering" in 2006. He was impressed by Indian engineers' ability to innovate cost-effectively and quickly, under severe resource constraints.

Here are five ways of frugal innovation; that is, achieving more with less:

1. **Eliminate:** a chain is made up of many small rings connected to each other. The more rings, the longer the distance between two ends of the chain. If eliminating some of the rings doesn't impact the use of the chain, such rings should be removed. For example, when a product is manufactured it goes through many hands in the distribution chain. The ultimate objective is to take the product to the end customer. If a manufacturer directly reaches the customer, it eliminates the distribution chain. Online shopping is a good example of the business-to-customer chain.

2. **Substitute:** finding or using substitutes is the best way to reduce costs. For example, loyalty programs have proven their benefits to the retail chains. Big retail chains can afford the cost of running the loyalty programs using software. Small retailers cannot afford this cost. Coffee shops in Sydney run loyalty programs using a small paper card. Every time a customer buys a coffee in the shop, the loyalty card is manually stamped. After getting the card stamped a certain number of times, the customer gets a free coffee.

3. **Combine:** combining more than one concept together helps to widen the customer base. The Tiffany show in Pattaya, Bangkok, is the best example. The Tiffany show is a combination of a play, music, a revolving stage, stunts, etc. The play also includes cultural dances on ten most popular languages, which helps to make the target customer segment broader.

4. **Add value:** adding more value to the existing product makes a huge difference. For example, the Commonwealth Bank of Australia launched "Card less Cash" using a mobile app. It is the same app that customers use to do basic transactions. The addition of cardless cash facility in the mobile app, gives customer more flexibility to withdraw cash without using card.

5. **Reuse:** reuse is a powerful tool. Mumbai Dabbawala, in India, launched a simple initiative to put a sticker on unused tiffins (lunchboxes) to redistribute them among the poor. This helped to save the waste of food as well as feed hungry people.

Frugal innovation is becoming more popular in the corporate world day by day. Organisations have understood the importance of doing more with less and going lean.

It's time to become lean in your personal life as well. Owning only what we need makes us flexible for change. It also helps to reduce attachment as we own less. After all, attachment is a root cause of stress.

Being creative is important

Think of our ancestors. When they were struggling to kill animals, they created tools. They were struggling so they became creative to solve the problem. If the problem cannot be solved by knowledge, the only way to find the solution is through creativity.

Creativity plays an important role in the corporate world. In a survey, where CEOs were asked about the most important skills, creativity took the topmost place in the list as a leadership skill. Creativity plays an important role in an organisation's survival as well. New products and new services play an important role in creating product differentiation, for which creativity is the base.

Earlier I talked about the consulting assignment I worked on, along with some of my colleagues, where the manager gave us two minutes to come up with a creative solution to a problem. I don't understand why some people think that creativity is operated like a button; you switch it on and you get creative. I have seen many forums where employees have been asked to give ideas within a day or so. What people fail to understand is that a mind full of thoughts cannot be creative.

Take the case of a pipe carrying water. As long as the pipe is full of water, nothing else can enter the pipe. So to fill the pipe with a new thing, first you need to empty it.

Many creative organisations work on these principles. The more creative the work environment, the more a feeling of relaxation is given to the employees. A relaxed mind is a creative mind and is more productive.

Research has proven that when employees are asked to find a solution to a complex problem in an offsite environment, more ideas are generated and of a better quality compared to when the same activity is done at the workplace. At the workplace, the mind is occupied with regular work-related activities, leaving little or no room for creativity.

If you observe anecdotal examples of Archimedes when he got his idea in the bathtub, or Newton when he got his idea under a tree, in both the cases they were in a relaxing environment. A writer goes away from urban life to a quiet place to finish their book, a painter finds an isolated place to finish their painting, a poet finds inspiration when in nature; all signify the importance of a relaxed mind.

While it is not always possible to have a relaxing environment in the corporate world, the ability to relax the mind under pressure helps us to remain creative.

To be creative you need to first let your existing thoughts go and empty the mind, and then acquire new knowledge. The only solution to struggle is creativity, which will find a way.

Creativity x Implementation = Innovation

Innovation is a product of creativity and implementation. You increase one of the elements and it will have a major impact on innovation.

Struggle -> Creativity-> Innovation

If you struggle, it means you are following the old ways of doing things. Use creativity to find new ways to avoid the struggle, which will lead to innovation. Creativity is the link between struggle and innovation.

Struggle can be avoided only by using creativity; that's how the world is evolving.

You need to be more creative every day.

Activity

Try this experiment in your workplace.

Ask participants to take a moment and draw a shape. Just a shape. Most people will draw a known shape, like a circle, rectangle or star.

Ask participants to relax, be quiet for few moments, walk around the room, then Google different shapes. Now ask them to draw a creative shape. You will experience a difference in the results.

I have conducted this experiment during my training sessions, and I have seen people, when relaxed, coming up with amazing shapes never seen before.

When you ask a kid, who is yet to learn shapes, to draw a shape, you will see that their shape will be unique because it doesn't come from a preconceived notion. The same principle applies when you empty the mind.

One of my friends visited me in Sydney recently and wanted to explore. He booked the City Tour. This didn't excite me as I am near all the places the tour visits almost every day because I work there. But then, it would have been inappropriate to ask my friend to go on his own. So I decided to join him and keep him company.

When I was taking the tour, I was surprised by the information that the tour guide shared. Most of the buildings were just buildings to me, but after the tour, I felt like many of these buildings and places became alive with historical events attached to them. I also walked many lanes that I never knew existed. At the end of the tour, I had a completely different perspective of the same area where I spent most of my time.

Stepping outside your normal pattern and seeing the world not just differently but with incredible openness is called divergent thinking. It's like walking in a garden with a toddler. Even if you try to drag the toddler, their curiosity will make them observe every little thing on the way. If you follow the toddler with their perspective, you will observe a completely different world.

That's how the term "walking in the customer's shoes" has evolved. You need to see the products and services from the customer's perspective. That's where creativity will play an important role when designing new products and services.

"To understand someone else's emotions, you need to walk in their shoes."

Have you done something wonderful? The story of an ant

It was a long queue. She had carried the food for a really long distance. She was an ant. She was about to reach the ant colony when she heard the question, "Have you done something wonderful in your life?"

She looked back. Her friend behind her had asked this question. She stopped for a moment. Suddenly, other ants behind her started shouting because she had stopped the whole queue and nobody was willing to jump the queue. She hurriedly moved ahead thinking that she had done many wonderful things, like she had cooked an amazing dish for her kids that morning, and last month she bought a really beautiful dress for her birthday. Wasn't that amazing? She decided to jot down all the wonderful things she'd done. She tried to remember all the wonderful things she had done in the last month, then in the last year, then in the last few years and then in her entire life. She then looked at the list and she felt as if her heart had stopped. She couldn't write down one thing that was really wonderful.

She said to herself, "I haven't done a single wonderful thing in my life. Then what have I done? Every day getting up, getting ready, following the queue to the food, collecting the food and bringing it to the colony. That's it! I am quite old now... Oh my God! I have just wasted my life! I don't know what's going to happen tomorrow, but I'm still alive and still have an opportunity do something wonderful."

She called her friends and explained to everyone why it was necessary to do something wonderful in their life. One of her friends shouted at her, "What wonderful thing can we do? We're ants. Are we going to build an aeroplane and fly? This is insane!"

Instead of getting demotivated, her friend's comments gave her an idea. "Yes!" she said, "We're ants and we're known for discipline. But we know how painful it is to follow the queue and collect the food. Can we do something about it? Can we break the queue and still bring the food?"

Everyone started laughing. Some of the ants hugged themselves while they laughed and started jumping. Ant felt embarrassed.

Then she suddenly shouted, "I have an idea. We can do something wonderful. What we need to do is just hug each other, collect the food and start jumping towards our colony. So we won't get bored and we will still do our work." There was pin-drop silence. Her friends liked her idea but didn't look convinced. "Or maybe we can just make a hollow ball by hugging each other and carry the food inside the ball to the colony, make the ball roll towards the colony. So we will be really fast and carry lots of food at a time. It'll be so much fun!"

The next day they tried the new technique and they collected enough food for the whole of the rainy reason. This made a difference to everyone's life in the colony. Ant now had something on her list and started thinking about what else could be done.

Do we need to learn only discipline from ants and form queues in front of the office entrance every morning, waiting to swipe our cards?

Monotony is the root cause of dullness. We don't feel energised going to the same place and doing the same thing day after day, year after year.

There is an important concept in marketing management related to the product lifecycle. A product follows a similar lifecycle to a human being.

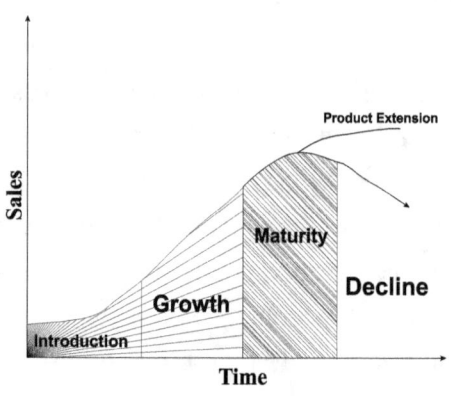

Fig.- Product life cycle

To delay the decline of a product, marketers use the concept of extending the product lifecycle. What this means is that when the product is at its peak and starts to decline, i.e., it starts to lose market share, changes are made so that it maintains or increases its market share instead. It could be a change in packaging, a promotion, etc. That's the important concept that can easily be used in the human lifecycle.

You will see many successful people doing something different at the peak of their career. Many get a feeling that they have hit a glass ceiling when they reach a certain level in the organisational hierarchy, and that's the time when you need to think about giving some extension to your excitement in life. Excitement will come from doing what you like, and you will get clarity about what you really like and what you really want to do when you spend some time with yourself. Do some introspection, let go of grudges, stress and anxiety and make some space in your mind to let ideas play and take shape.

"Do something wonderful in life."

A man was walking through a dense jungle. He noticed it was deadly silent. Suddenly, he saw lots of monkeys in the trees around him. There were hundreds. The man was scared for a moment but decided not to show any reaction on his face. He continued his journey. All of a sudden, the monkeys started whooping and screeching. It was scarier than before. The man, still scared, continued his journey.

A huge monkey jumped down in front of the man. This was the scariest moment for the man and he thought maybe it was the end of his life. To his surprise, the monkey started talking to him.

"I appreciate your courage. We could not scare you."

There was a silence for some time as the man could not believe that the monkey was talking to him.

Monkey: "Who are you and where are you going?"
Man: "I am a human being and I am in search of something new."
Monkey: "I am the king of monkeys. I am the wisest creature on the Earth. I know everything. Ask me what you are looking for and I will give you information about it."

Man: "I'm looking for something that is not seen by the world."

Monkey: "There is nothing that is not seen by the world."

Man: "How do you know that?"

Monkey: "I'm not an ordinary monkey. I have a superpower."

The monkey jumped to the tallest branch of a tree, jumped from one tree to another, climbed another tree like a squirrel, hopped from one place to another and then came back to the man.

Monkey: "Didn't I tell you that I'm not an ordinary creature! I have seen the whole world."

Man was puzzled and didn't know how to react.

Man: "Have you been to the end of the world?"

Monkey: "Yes."

Man: "Can you go there for me one more time and tell me where exactly it is?"

Monkey: "Here I go."

Monkey took his longest jump for days, months, years. Finally, he reached a spot where he saw something similar to the man he had met. So he thought that it could be the end of the world. He decided to turn back, then suddenly realised that he needed to do something to prove that he had been to the end of the world. So he went to the man and tried lifting him on his shoulders to carry him along. Man started shouting, asking him why he was doing that. Monkey realised that he was the same man with whom he had met before. Monkey realised his mistake. There is no end to the world.

There is always an opportunity to find out something new or to do something new.

Man continued his journey.

What you see is not always true

It was the end of the day and I was preparing a nice Indian curry. There was little salt left in the jar, so I picked up a new packet from the cupboard and poured it into the jar. I added the usual quantity of salt to the curry. After some time, while it was still cooking, I tested the curry. It tasted like it didn't have any salt. So I added some more salt. Still I couldn't taste the salt in the curry. I added a good amount of salt and thought maybe some ingredient was causing sweetness. I cooked and ate curry like that. But somehow I was thinking about what had happened. Had I stopped being able to taste salt? I was worried. I took a pinch from the jar and tasted it. It was sugar. No wonder I couldn't taste salt in the curry. I realised my mistake as there was no way I could differentiate the salt and sugar. Both looked exactly the same. Then I had another challenge. There was some salt left at the bottom of the jar and I had filled sugar on top of it. How would I separate the sugar and salt?

We come across similar situations in life where it's difficult to differentiate between good and bad. Selecting good is like trying to select sugar from salt. It is difficult but not impossible. In the case of sugar and salt, salt is not soluble in alcohol, while sugar is. When you add the alcohol to the mixture, you can take out salt, then letting alcohol evaporate will give you sugar.

Just like you have to add alcohol to the mixture of salt and sugar to separate them, you have to add yogic practices to your life to separate good from bad.

Having a beautiful mind
"Who you work with has lots of influence on who you become."

I had a manager once who used the word frustration in almost every interaction. Whether he spoke about work, a person or anything, not only in the organisation but outside the organisation as well, he was always frustrated with everything. I even found a couple of his social media posts with the word frustration in them. I was frustrated with his frustration! But then I also started believing that the word "frustration" must be an influential word to use to get things done.

After getting really frustrated with my manager's frustration, I changed my job. The new organisation changed my perception and taught me the exact opposite. This organisation had just started a new business and was expanding like anything. So, of course, there was lots of pressure on us to launch new products as soon as possible. When there is huge pressure to meet deadlines, you will see lots of frustration around you. I became part of that frustration.

In after-hours' meetings, heated arguments had become a daily routine. But one person always carried a smile on his face, and that was the president of my business vertical. I thought perhaps it was because of his education from one of the top schools. I envied his calmness at his level. I decided to have a chat with him over a cup of tea. I wasn't sure whether my request would be entertained or not but I was hopeful as we were still a small team of roughly twenty-five people. His secretary took my request and, to my surprise, I got the fifteen-minute timeslot on a Friday morning in his diary.

On the day, I went to his office. He greeted me with a big smile and said, "Would you mind having a cup of tea outside the office?" I was delighted.

Over a cup of tea, we discussed some general topics and then he asked me, "What's bothering you?"

Bravely I asked, "How do you always maintain a smile on your face in such a stressful environment?" I was expecting an answer to do with some business model or concept.

He said, "I always want to have a beautiful mind."

Now this was surprising for me. He explained, "What you speak has a deep impact on your mind and thought process. If you are angry and try to vent that anger on someone else, or speak negatively, it has more negative impact on you than the other person because your mind is processing that interaction. However, it's highly impossible for us not to get angry in a corporate environment. So there is a little trick. Whenever you see your colleagues, always smile, even if you've had an argument with them, even if the next person doesn't respond with a smile. Make it a habit. Every day, whenever you see a colleague, greet them with a smile, forgetting your last interaction with that person."

This one simple habit has helped me to conquer many interactions. The very fact of a smile without any prejudice has helped me to understand the meaning of having a beautiful mind.

A beautiful mind cannot be described; it has to be experienced.

We need to talk

It was the month of December and I was travelling in New Zealand. I was in a hotel facing a lake in Queenstown. It was around seven in the evening and the sun was still bright. I had returned from a five-hour difficult hike and was tired as hell. I was drinking coffee just to feel alive and was looking at the beauty of the lake in front of me with a snow-capped mountain behind it, and tourists were busy taking photographs around the lake.

"We need to talk." I heard this from a gentleman sitting close to me. For a moment I was surprised as I thought he was talking to me. But when I looked at him he was alone at his table and there was a bottle of liquor in front of him. He was holding a glass of liquor poured from the bottle. And he was looking at the bottle and talking to the bottle. Well, it was an interesting scene. Not a rare one though.

He continued, "We're dating a lot since the time I lost my job two months back. We see each other every day. You make me happy... um really... let me think... Do you really make me happy? Honestly, I don't know... you actually taste like shit... Actually shit. So your taste doesn't make me happy. But when I drink you, I feel happy... um, actually I don't feel sad. So I think you don't make me happy but you just help me to forget my sadness... you are such a sweetheart. Thank you for that. That really helps me. I forget my sadness. Hooray! Hey, but hang on, you come with a problem... I can't drive after drinking you! And, and do you remember last time I drank in a hotel and said something to the bar attendant, I was almost arrested for misbehaviour... Hmm, that's not a good thing. And, hey, one more thing, you make me forget sadness only when I'm drunk. When I get up in the morning, you just leave me back in my original state. The sadness returns. This is not fair. If I'm loyal to you, you should be loyal to me. But you're not. You are so selfish, I hate you."

He stared at the bottle in anger for a minute or so. Suddenly, he picked up the bottle and threw it in the trash. Then he said, "I should try drugs." And he disappeared. I felt sad for that guy. He was clearly struggling with job loss and was depressed. Anyway, I continued with my dinner.

The next morning when I entered the restaurant, this guy was drinking tea and looking at the beautiful lake and snow-capped mountains. He looked relaxed. I wished him a good morning. He asked me to join him. I was a little uncomfortable, but still I joined him. We spoke about our travels. And then I reminded him about his last statement from the previous day that he would try drugs. I politely suggested that he should not do that. The thought of recent deaths of youngsters at music festivals in Australia ran through my mind for a second. He smiled and replied, "Oh, don't worry, I was too drunk last night and I would never try drugs in my life. In fact, I've quit drinking from today."

I laughed loudly as I'd heard this from so many of my friends many times over, and then seen them go back to drinking again. He realised why I laughed, so he smiled and said, "No, I'm serious. And the reason is that when I drink, I forget about everything for some time. It doesn't mean I'm happy, it's just that I forget the reality about myself and things around me and I mistake it as happiness. In fact, when I'm not under the influence of alcohol, I come back to reality and then I find it more difficult to handle the reality. So I go back to drinking again to forget the reality. The solution is not to forget the reality for some time but to make myself capable of facing it and be stronger to handle the reality."

"That's a good idea," I said. "But how will you do that? Just curious."

He said, "I'll try yoga and meditation. I've heard a lot about it. I don't know if it'll help or not. But no harm in trying. Let's see."

I wished him good luck and said goodbye, and thanked him for sowing that seed of beautiful thought in my mind as well.

Bringing the broken pieces together

When I was a child, we used to live in a village. My sister was sent to my uncle's house in another district for her high school education as our village didn't have a high school. One Diwali, my sister visited us, and after the celebration was over, she had to go back to the district place. I wanted to go with my beloved sister, and I kept nagging her a couple of days before her departure. Just to avoid my disappointment, everyone promised me I could go. When the day came for her departure, I accompanied her to the bus stop along with my dad. The bus came, my sister boarded the bus, but I was pulled aside. I was surprised, my eyes filled with tears and I felt like I'd been cheated. I was crying loudly, and using all my strength to get out of my father's grip so I could board the bus. The bus left. I saw my sister's face with tears rolling down her cheeks, sadly waving at me.

I was really mad and felt cheated. I didn't like anyone as everyone around me had lied to me. I was so disturbed that I wanted to hit everyone around me for cheating me and breaking their promise. I was sad for the whole day. The next day I was still angry. My mother kept an empty clay pot to serve breakfast. I picked up the pot and threw it at the wall and it broke immediately. My mother was really angry but she knew my emotions so she didn't say anything. I refused to go to school.

My father, who would never tolerate missing school, didn't say anything. He asked me to get ready and promised to take me out. Reluctantly, I took a bath and joined him. He took me to a potter's house. The potter used to make beautiful things and used to gift some to us out of great respect for my father. He asked the potter to explain the process of making a pot. I realised that it was a distraction, and I didn't want to learn anything. But the potter was so loving. He pulled me into his arms, kissed my cheek and offered me some biscuits. And he said to my father to leave me with him. My father left.

The potter took me into his backyard where he was digging soil for making earthen pots. He told me that we would make a nice toy. First he told me you need the clay. Mixing clay and water and then making a mound out of it was a wonderful process. I enjoyed it. After making the mound, he took a small ball off the mound and put it on the wheel and asked me to rotate it as fast as I could. My little hands put all my force into it and I tried to rotate the wheel. I wasn't strong enough so he helped me. As soon as the wheel started rotating, he kept the mound at the centre of the wheel and started giving it shape.

The mound slowly turned into an object. Every touch changed its appearance. I, too, started giving it some shape. It was fun. At the end, there was a beautiful tiny earthen pot with my fingerprints on it. Yay! We were both happy. The potter picked up that delicate earthen pot from the centre of the wheel and kept it aside. I insisted he give it to me. But then he showed me how delicate it was and how it would be destroyed by the time I reached home. I didn't want to destroy it as I felt I'd created that. He asked me to leave it in the sun for two days.

This whole incident took more than an hour. My father came back, and I was a little less angry. The potter asked me to come back after two days. I eagerly waited for the two days to be over to go and get the pot. On the third day I went to see my pot. It was hard and beautiful. I asked if I could take it home. The potter said, "You can, but it won't last long."

I said I wanted to use it as a piggy bank to collect money to visit my sister. So he told me we needed to make it stronger. They call the process burning, wherein they put the pots close to the fire. He took my pot and put it in the special oven made for burning these kinds of pots. He asked me to wait for some time. The potter turned the pot every now and then to make sure it was heated equally on all sides. He did this for all the pots in the oven. It was a tedious job as he had to go close to the oven to turn the pots. His face was covered with ash and sweat, but his face did not show any complaint. I felt pity for him for what he had to go through.

Finally, after an hour or so, he pulled my pot out of the oven and put it on the ground. It looked more beautiful now. After he said it was finished, the potter cleaned it with a cloth and the pot started shining. It was my pot. He handed it over to me and gave me a hug. I hurriedly rushed home. I showed it to all on my way saying I had made it, with pride to attract jealous eyes from my friends. My parents were equally happy. My father pulled me closer. He showed me the broken pieces of the pot that I had broken in anger. He asked, "Now do you realise what you have done?" Confused with his question I looked at his face. He took the pot from my hand and said, "Look how beautiful this is. But how much you had to put into it to make it. Now if someone breaks it in a second, how would you feel?" I realised my mistake. My father said, "We take lots of pains to make something but a small dose of anger can destroy it completely." I looked at the broken pieces of the pot and felt really sorry.

This whole episode played in my mind when I recently visited one of my Japanese friend's houses. She had a beautiful pot that she'd broken inadvertently but had tried to fix by bringing all the pieces together with a golden-coloured glue. It looked so cute. She explained to me the concept of kintsugi. There is a belief in their society that breaking things is a bad omen. But sometimes it can happen inadvertently. While many cultures talk about leaving things behind if they're broken, the Japanese philosophy gives importance to rebuilding the broken pieces, as a lot of effort has gone into building it. They call this kintsugi.

I really like this concept, because the hardships we face shape who we are. Just like someone who has survived a war and has scars on their body treats it as a symbol of tenacity and the fighting attitude of a soldier; similarly, scars that we feel from heartbreak, loss, betrayal or disappointment are part of our history and our stories about survival. Rather than hiding them, kintsugi encourages us to celebrate them.

Kintsugi is finding joy in imperfections and celebrating them.

Change management—why so difficult?

"It is not the strongest of the species that survive, nor the most intelligent, but the most responsive to change." —Charles Darwin

We are new every day. Even the way we look changes every day. Millions of cells die every day and millions of new cells are born. We are never the same, so why do we try to be the same? That's where one of the fundamentals of change lies.

One of the most challenging tasks for an organisation is to manage change. This becomes more challenging for multinational organisations because of the differences in cultures. Change management professionals use practices such as ADKAR to address change. ADKAR represents the five outcomes that people need to achieve for lasting change, which are:

1. **A**wareness
2. **D**esire

3. **K**nowledge
4. **A**ttitude
5. **R**einforcement

Despite such practices, many organisations still face problems during the implementation of change.

"There is only one thing that is constant and that is change."

This saying is quite old, but still organisations face change-related problems. The worst thing that can happen in organisations is people who resist change. They suffer more and, at the end of the day, most of the planned changes take place anyway.

So it becomes a win–win situation to accept change. Change is about changing the current state. Change management is all about handling resistance to change, which is like trying to stop water from moving.

Confucius said, *"Flowing water never stagnates and the hinges of an active door never rust. This is due to movement. The same principle applies to essence and energy. If the body does not move, essence does not flow, energy stagnates."*

This is true in the corporate world, too. If you do not change, you will be left behind.

So change is good. It opens doors to new opportunities.

An individual's resistance to change could be because of:

- perceived insecurity
- being out of their comfort zone
- fear of the unknown.

It is interesting to know where these three factors come from. They come from belief. And where do these beliefs come from? Every belief has a fragment of thought and every thought is related to some past experience. So our beliefs are based on our experiences from the past. Our beliefs make us live in the past. Living in the past restricts our growth. The moment we challenge our own beliefs, we open our minds to welcome new changes.

Just like stored water can become stagnant over a period of time, beliefs can also become poisonous for our growth.

Yogis do not fear change. In fact, yogis are open to change and they look forward to change because they believe that "to be soft and flexible is the way of life and to be hard and rigid is the way to death".

You will see the stagnated careers of many who've resisted change, and they will remain in the same situation for years. On the contrary, those who embrace change will experience a new life with every new change. The expansion is human nature. Expansion of knowledge, expansion of territory, expansion of skills, etc. Those who don't want to expand create a boundary around themselves and become their own prisoners. Someone else putting you in prison is one thing; you creating your own prison is another. You creating your own prison is more dangerous than someone putting you in prison. When you resist change, you block the opportunity of expansion and create your own prison.

Accept and adjust with the change.

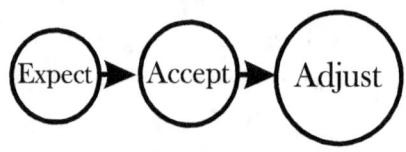

Fig.- Accepting the change

"Do not fear with change; be like water."

Water was travelling along its way. It believed in flowing, and if there were obstacles in its way, it bypassed them but didn't stop moving. One day, Water met a huge rock. They soon became good friends. But Rock was arrogant. It had been there for thousands of years, still in the same form and shape. Rock told all these beautiful stories of staying in one place. Rock told Water the benefits of staying in one place. "Since you are in one place, there are better chances of survival and you'll live longer, you will observe all the beautiful seasons from one place, and no one will bother you." Water was convinced with what Rock was saying and decided to stay in the one place.

Water was there for some time and it became stagnant and started stinking. Lots of bacteria grew inside it and it was evaporating. Water realised that it wasn't its nature to stay in one place, but should remain flexible and keep moving.

Water started running. This didn't make Rock happy, and Rock started chasing Water. While running, both fell off a cliff edge of a high mountain. Water became a beautiful waterfall and also helped to generate power, while Rock was broken into pieces. Broken Rock was carried away by Water into the ocean. The broken pieces went to the bottom of the ocean and were never seen again. When Water merged with the ocean it merged with the waves and shined.

Even the fall of water is beautiful. If a rock falls it breaks, but when water falls it generates power and looks beautiful. Being obsessed with yourself is like being a rock; being flexible is like being water.

Bruce Lee's famous quote says: "You must be shapeless, formless, like water. When you pour water in a cup, it becomes the cup. When you pour water in a bottle, it becomes the bottle. When you pour water in a teapot, it becomes the teapot. Water can drip and it can crash. Become like water, my friend."

I was so impressed with the sound of djembe drumming that I wanted to learn it myself. One of my friend's, Eyal, from Israel, gave me a lesson. After practising the rhythm for a couple of days, I felt like I had already become a master of djembe. I decided to play in the drum circle. Excited, I started playing, and I followed exactly the rhythm taught to me, but something was wrong. I could feel the look "You are new" from the people around me. I couldn't understand what I was doing wrong. During the break, Eyal came to me with a smile and took my djembe between his knees.

He said, "My friend, music is not playing the same rhythm. Music is creating a variation. We start with variation, what we normally say 'Call' at the start, then we use the variation at certain intervals to break the rhythm, and then we use variation again at the end. That makes the music. To create the music you need to create the variation in the rhythm."

If even melodious music is a result of change, then how can we resist change in the work environment? In fact, if there is no change, we should seek the change.

FDI model of relationships

Relationships are such complex things that they can be difficult to explain. While modern behavioural science struggles to explain the basis of a relationship, yogic practices explain them effortlessly.

Through the lens of yogic practices, a relationship can be understood through the FDI model, where any relationship is the result of one or a combination of the following factors:

- **F**eelings; for example, love.
- **D**eficiency; for example, the employee–employer relationship.
- **I**nfluence; for example, the teacher and student, the politician and the public.

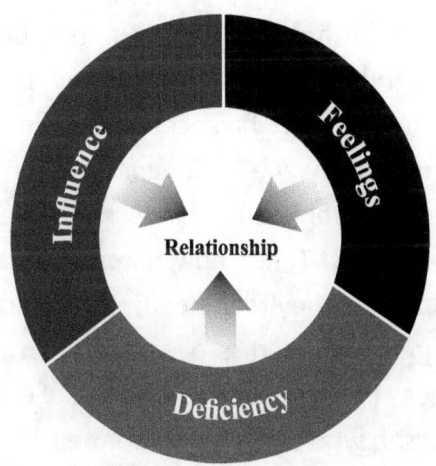

Fig.- FDI model of relationship

Feelings: if you have some feelings for someone, then that creates the relationship. If you like someone, you may fall in love, which gives rise to the relationship. Even being blood relations does not carry any meaning in the absence of feelings. Two brothers separated in childhood will not feel any relationship until they realise that they are brothers and develop that feeling. Brotherly love and a relationship will originate from that feeling. Similarly, two people known to each other and who have a blood relationship will not have a relationship in the

203

absence of feelings. When the feelings are over, for whatever reason, the relationship breaks down.

If someone wants love, you should give them love. What we need to understand is that no one wants hatred.

Deficiency: when we have a vitamin deficiency we take vitamin tablets to re-establish the balance in the body. Similarly, if someone is in need of something, they need to get that something to maintain the balance in their life. If we no longer suffer from a deficiency, we no longer need the help of vitamin tablets. Similarly, if people don't have any shortage they may not go back to the source. That's how nature works. So if someone takes your help when they're in need, that person may not come back to you once the need is over; we term it as selfishness. What we forget is that that's how nature works. The way this applies to a person who came to you for help, also applies to you as well. Tomorrow, you may take someone's help and then forget that person afterwards. It's just that we may not realise that we also act selfishly. So we call the whole world selfish. It is true. What creates the problem is when we don't accept it. And when the whole world is selfish, we are also part of it.

Influence: when a leader is elected, he/she is the result of their influence over the masses. That influence creates a leader–follower relationship. A true leader is one who respects their followers. If someone comes to you because of your influence, you should love them even more.

"The problem is not winning friends and people, the problem is retaining them."

People will lose feelings, people will be selfish, we will be selfish, and we will lose our influence. All these things follow the cycle. If we do not accept these facts and hate people, hatred will bring frustration. When we are frustrated, we are the biggest losers.

A good understanding of this model will help to solve many behavioural issues at work.

Take a real break

"Ah! It's Monday again." This is a common thing to hear on a Monday morning. The Monday blues is a popular phrase to describe this phenomenon. The weekend is always too short. In fact, even a week-long break seems short. When we return from a holiday, it feels like the time passed very fast. Many times we expect a good break on the holiday but sometimes it doesn't seem like a break at all. The reason is, in reality, we don't get a break.

At the end of a day's work we feel tired. Even if we work sitting in one place, we still feel tired because we've used our mental capacity. But at the same time, even if we don't do anything throughout the day, we feel tired. The brain is to blame. Even if we don't do anything, the brain is still working and sometimes thinking hard about something, which makes us feel tired. The same thing happens over the weekend. Even if we don't do anything, the mind is still at work, and when we come back to

205

work on Monday, we don't feel like we've had a rest. Similarly, when we go on vacation, our mind is still working. The worst thing is if you keep thinking about work during the weekend or during your vacation, then it definitely doesn't count as a break.

When we hit the bed at the end of the day we need to rest. If we can't sleep properly at night, we feel weak and lethargic throughout the next day. Taking a break is the key. If we are doing a physical activity, we take a break every now and then because the body becomes tired. Similarly, the mind needs a break, too.

The definition of a sprint is a "run at full speed over a short distance". You can't run at a high speed for a long time. This concept is borrowed by the corporate world in software development. Traditionally, software development followed the cycle of gathering all the software requirements at once and then developing the whole software and delivering it. Sometimes this development took months to complete, and things could change during this period resulting in a change in requirement. Many times, issues in the requirement were identified at the end of development, resulting in software features being completely different to the requirement. The software industry came up with the agile concept in which the whole work is divided into small chunks of deliverables, most of the time with a two-week time span. This helps to deliver the features regularly while the development is still ongoing.

Retrospection is an important part of this methodology. Team members gather at the end of each delivery and retrospect about what went wrong and what went well, and the necessary actions are taken if things did not go to plan in the previous delivery. So, essentially, they take a small pause to reflect, and then go again at full speed to deliver the next deliverable; that's why they call it a sprint.

We need to practise sprint or pause in our life as well.

A pause gives you an opportunity to calm down, collect your energy and do the next activity with full force. Unfortunately, we often don't get that pause on the weekends or on holidays because the mind is still working at the same speed as it was working in the office. Give the mind a pause every now and then. Make it empty and you will rejuvenate it automatically.

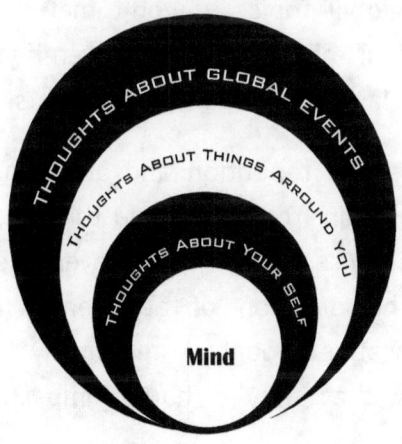

Fig.- Layers of thoughts

When you meditate, all the thoughts that come into your mind can be divided into different layers.

The outer layer—global events—are things that are happening in the world, country, city, etc. Upon realising that we haven't seen what's going on or if we don't think of these events for some time, there is no harm; we can stop getting these thoughts. The next layer is thoughts about work, family and things that directly affect you. It takes a good amount of effort to convince ourselves that it is in our best interest not to think about these things, even for a few minutes. The next layer is new thoughts that the mind starts contemplating or thoughts about yourself; this is a similar state to daydreaming. With constant practise, these thoughts can also be minimised.

Just like it's easier to convince ourselves that even if we stop thinking about global topics it won't matter, similarly, after regular practise, our mind realises that even if you stop thinking about the middle layer and inner layer thoughts, it won't matter.

Yogic life is all about repetition and abstinence. When yogis meditate, they abstain from unwanted things for the period of the meditation. They repeat this during every meditation. Slowly they increase the duration of abstinence (especially from unwanted or negative thoughts) and finally they become so strong internally that they're hardly impacted by negative thoughts.

Yogic life vs a non-yogic life

Yogic life	Non-yogic life
Vegetables	Meat
Yoga	Exercise
Alkaline food	Acidic food
Harmony	Competition
Belonging	Privacy
Relations (equal importance to others)	Strong personal identity
Collectivism	Individualism
Love	Hatred
Union of mind–body–soul	Lack of coordination between mind, body and soul
Focus on achieving consciousness	Lack of consciousness
Focus on ultimate joy	Focus on momentary happiness

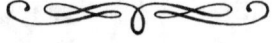

Chapter 4

Yogic healing

"Not every treatment comes from a bottle of pills."

As discussed in chapter one of this book, there are five major external factors causing stress. Yogic solutions to these stress causing factors are as below-

Factor	Yogic Solution
The pain of separation from loved ones	Detachment
The pain of losing wealth	Awareness
Fear of losing wealth	Positive attitude
Insulting words	Understanding ego
FOMO- fear of missing out	Creativity

Yoga journey discussed in chapter two helps to reduce the effect of these external factors causing stress.

Self-healing

Healing can be divided into two major types:

1. Healing from the outside.
2. Healing from the inside.

Self-healing is healing from the inside. It is the most powerful healing. It almost sounds mysterious—how would we heal ourselves? When you feel sad, you don't stay sad forever. You come out of sadness. That is the self-healing power of your body. When you get bruises on your body, and even if you don't do anything, your body has the power to heal automatically. Blood will clot on its own and bruises will stop bleeding. You sit down quietly and your heart rate goes down, your blood pressure becomes normal. Our body knows how to heal; it's just that we need to trust our body.

We all think that when we become ill, medicines will cure the illness. Medicines don't cure the illness, rather, they just accelerate the function of the body to cure itself. Just like medicine accelerates the healing process, yoga and medicine also do the same thing. Modern medicines have the capability to accelerate the process rapidly, but they often come with side effects.

On the contrary, if you stimulate your body in the wrong way, it can harm itself. If you are tense, your blood pressure rises, your muscles tense, you don't breathe properly, and so on.

It is important to have the awareness that your body listens to you. There are countless examples where people have recovered from incurable diseases, just because of their will power. No matter what you are suffering from, let your body know that you love it and will pay attention to it. Help your body to recover from whatever it is suffering from. Give the love to your body that it deserves.

Try a simple experiment. Whenever you feel lonely or stressed, try to massage your head with your hands, gently as if your mother is touching your head and showing love. Hug yourself. Treat your body as if you are a mother and your body is your child. Take deep breaths. If you have made a mistake, try not to be too hard on yourself. Mistakes happen. Hug yourself. Give that much-needed hug to your body. Your body needs your attention.

If you've had a bad day, try avoiding repetitive, negative thoughts. Listen to music. Meditate. Laugh, dance and sing. Enjoy your own company. The body already knows how to heal and live happily, we just need to avoid creating an obstacle in the healing process.

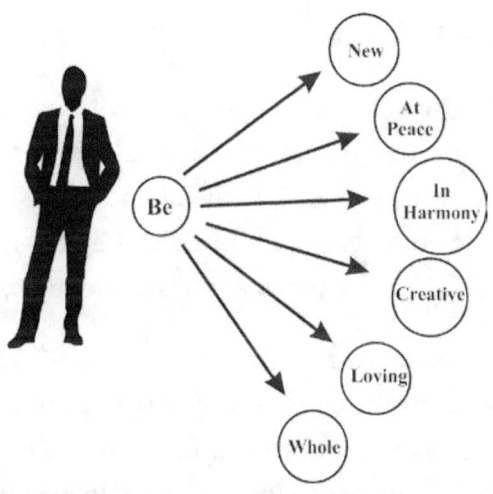

Fig.-Self Healing

Self-healing organisations

A self-healing organisation is one that is not dependent on others for addressing its problems. Hiring consultants to address problems is a common practice in organisations. This costs a huge amount of money, plus organisations become dependent on external parties. Self-healing organisations are about building the capability within the organisation so that whenever there are problems they can be addressed internally. A self-healing organisation is an efficient organisation as there is awareness among all to pick up the small problems and address them before they become big, thus taking care of employees and stakeholders and, ultimately, customers.

Healing through breath

In 1931, Dr Otto Warburg received the Nobel Prize for his discovery that low oxygen was characteristic of cancer cells. The primary condition associated with all forms of cancer is the severe deficiency of oxygen to the cells of affected tissues, and cancer cannot occur in tissues that are sufficiently oxygenated.

Supplying sufficient oxygen to the cells is the best way to prevent cancer, and the best way to supply sufficient oxygen to the cells is pranayama. Pranayama not only prevents but cures many ailments by supplying extra oxygen. Uneven breathing is a symptom of stress. Conscious, even, deep breathing reduces stress, preventing stress-related disorders.

Your lifespan is not measured by the number of years but by the number of breaths you take.

In the ancient story of the tortoise and the hare, the hare ran faster and took faster breaths, while the tortoise was slower but finished the race first. Corporate life is full of hares; they are just running. In fact, the majority of them are running with only short-term goals in sight, such as getting a salary hike, getting a new job or getting a promotion. Many can't finish the race and finish in between the goals.

The correlation between the number of breaths versus the average lifespan is shown below-

	Approx. number of breaths per minute	Average lifespan expectancy
Hare	55	10
Human being	15–18	70
Tortoise	3–5	193

When you are in bed relaxing, you will realise that your breath has slowed down. It can change quickly if you suddenly think of danger; it gets faster. Slow breath is a sign of relaxation. A relaxed body and mind help to maintain the flow of energy to all parts of the body. Any sort of tension immediately reduces the flow of energy.

During the day, our breath is on autopilot mode. It is affected by external factors, such as emotions and thoughts. Whenever breath is affected it impacts the flow of energy. *The Yellow Emperor's Classic of Internal Medicine* states: "Anger causes energy to rise, joy causes energy to slow, grief causes energy to dissipate, fear causes energy to descend, fright causes energy to shatter, exhaustion causes energy to wither, worry causes energy to stagnate."

Whenever you feel that you have irregular breath, even if you're not doing any physically straining work, a conscious effort to regulate your breath will help to reduce the impact of emotional imbalance.

The best way to slow your breath is to sit quietly in a quiet place and observe the breath. If possible, lie on your back with your eyes closed. Keep both your hands near the naval region. Feel the inflation and deflation of the naval region with every breath. Concentrate on the movement and the flow of air in and out of your body. Meditation slows down the breath.

Breathing pace	What it means
Less than 5 seconds a breath	When you notice this, try to be quiet and slow down the breath.
10 seconds a breath	This is a sign of relaxation.
15–20 seconds a breath	This is sign that you are calm and relaxed.
30–60 seconds a breath	You are in meditation.
90 seconds a breath	You are in deep meditation.
Towards samadhi	Slower breaths will help you to achieve samadhi.
The masters	As a result of samadhi, many masters are able to hold their breath for longer.

People talk about lung cleansing drinks or food. In reality, proper breath is the biggest healer, not only for the lungs but for all organs of the body. All organs need oxygen to function properly as every organ is made up of cells. Supplying enough oxygen to rejuvenate the cells of the body helps to heal the respective organs.

Our breath changes with our emotions. Different emotions will have a different impact on the breath.

- When you are scared, the breath will be a little faster.
- When you are anxious, the breath will be short and shallow, mostly from the top of the lungs.
- When you are angry your breath has jerks and pauses; breath keeps shifting between the nose and the mouth.
- Fear causes long retention of breath, or shallow breathing.
- When you are sad, your breath is shallow, slow and sometimes comes to a complete halt.
- When you are happy, your breath is deeper and long.
- When you are calm, your breath is slow, long and deep.

Based on breathing patterns, you can recognise the emotional state of yourself or the people around you. Emotional imbalances cause irregular breathing, which deprives the body of much-needed oxygen, resulting in damage to vital internal organs.

Depending on what type of emotional state you are in, you can often alter your emotional state using proper breathing techniques and helping your body and mind to recover from the imbalance.

Ancient alternate medicines give great importance to the healing power of breath. The Taoism philosophy of Chinese origin gives great importance to breathing techniques. There is a separate section in Taoist philosophy called "Tuna", which roughly translates as spitting (muddy) and receiving (clean).

Healing through meditation

We carry so many toxins in our mind in the form of memories and feelings. We allow certain feelings and emotions to have a permanent place in our mind and we carry them with us as part of our character. Meditation helps to empty the mind. When you empty the mind, you also empty the toxins of memory.

Levels of stress:

If you wave your hands on the surface of water, it creates a disturbance on the surface of the water, but the impact of this disturbance reduces as you go deeper into the water. If the water is really deep, the impact of the disturbance on the surface may not reach the bottom at all. On the contrary, if there is an impact at the bottom, it will always travel upward, as that is the only direction it can go. Earthquakes at the bottom of the ocean cause tsunamis; air released at the bottom of an aquarium bubbles to the top.

Emotions also have similar effects. If the emotions touch deep inside us, they will have a big impact. Stronger the mind; lesser the impact.

When we meditate, we go deep inside ourselves, thus cleansing the emotions deep within us. You might remember the worst things that have happened to you or the best things while in meditation. You may have tears rolling down your cheeks or a big smile on your face. During meditation, you go deep inside to take care of the mind. This helps to erase negative impressions on your mind, healing your mind.

When you're stressed and feeling miserable, you watch a comedy movie, which acts as a distraction and you forget about your worries. You speak to a friend, family member, you read an interesting book, sing, dance, etc. All these activities make you concentrate on something else, bringing steadiness of mind that relieves you from the distress and helps the healing process. So anything that facilitates concentration and inward absorption is meditative and is going to help you heal.

"We have been looking at causes of diseases and now it is obvious that 95% of all chronic inflammation in the body is connected to heart disease, cancer and even Alzheimer's. There is inflammation in the body, inflammation in the brain, inflammation in the immune system, and when people practise meditation, mindfulness, awareness, the inflammation in the body comes down and with compassion, love, kindness, joy, inflammation also comes down, which helps to heal the body."

—Deepak Chopra during one of his interactions with His holiness Dalai Lama.

Inflammation is the body's response to protect itself in certain situations, such as injuries and infection. Chronic inflammation is when the body is in a constant state of alert. Over a period of time, chronic inflammation can have a serious, negative impact on the body. Some of the symptoms of chronic inflammation include fatigue, low mood, unexplained aches and stomach problems. Chronic stress is considered as one of the main causes of chronic inflammation, along with unhealthy food, smoking and alcohol.

Meditation helps to relax the body and mind. A relaxed body and mind helps to reduce the stress, which results in a reduction of chronic inflammation. Someone who suffers from high blood pressure, and has used a 24-hour blood pressure monitoring device, will tell you that their blood pressure drops drastically during the night when they are asleep, as the body is relaxed. It has been observed that blood pressure drops when you meditate. So there is a visible effect of meditation. A regular meditation practice not only helps to reduce inflammation (heal) but also helps to prevent illness (by controlling unwanted inflammation).

Healing though yoga

Yoga is not a fashion, luxury or spirituality, it is a natural way to maintain health and achieve happiness.

In yoga, you generate your own energy to fight diseases.

In yoga, there are three types of disorders:

1. Self-inflicted: if we abuse our bodies, we will have to pay the price for it.

2. Congenital disease: those that you suffer on account of your genes.
3. Diseases because of imbalance: caused by an imbalance of the five elements in our system.

There are different scales to measure the different physical aspects of the human body. A weighing scale measures weight, a thermometer measures temperature. These scales tell you where you stand with respect to normal measurement. We take action based on the reading of these scales. Unfortunately, there is no such scale for the functioning of the mind.

Yogic literature classifies the different states of mind, which can be treated as a scale:

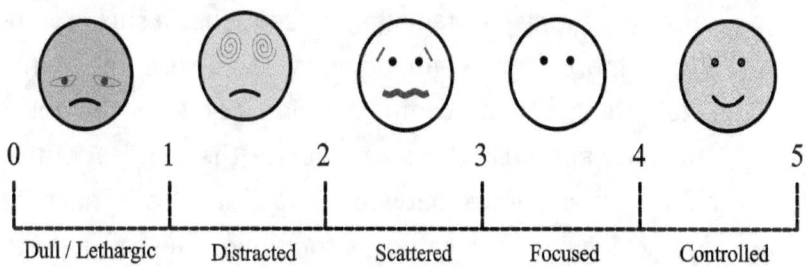

Fig.-States of mind

All these above states are like a scale. We fit into one of the states, while the severity may vary from person to person depending on the situation. The objective is to move from left to right on this scale. Looking at this scale you can decide what mental state you are in, and take action accordingly. Yoga helps to improve the state of mind.

- **Dull/lethargic:** this state of mind is normally because of some loss, traumatic experience, etc. Dullness causes loss of appetite, concentration and sleep. A person in this state is disinclined to observe, act or react. This is rarely a permanent situation but in many cases it could last longer depending on the severity of loss or experience. Yoga gradually reduces the symptoms by relaxing the mind. Regular practise will lead to the transformation of negative energy into positive energy.
- **Distracted:** lack of decision-making ability, confusion, feeling lost and having unclear goals are the symptoms of this state. It arises because of flawed signals from the senses, creating contradicting perceptions. In such a state it is important to calm down and stabilise the mind. Establishing proper communication between the mind and the senses can help to stabilise the mind. A stable mind can separate between good and bad, right or wrong. Staying in yoga poses for some time can help to focus and concentrate and will bring calmness.
- **Scattered:** this state of mind is because of a lack of confidence and fear. A fearful mind cannot succeed. Yoga practice can bring optimism, clarity of thoughts, boost confidence and reduce fear.

- **Focused:** a focused mind is an undisturbed mind. Such a mind has concentration and confidence. A focused mind is a stable mind with clarity.
- **Controlled:** a controlled mind is the highest state of mind where the mind has control over itself. Sensory organs cannot dominate such a mind. A controlled mind experiences joy, as external factors cannot affect it.

Healing through sound

Ever wondered how people battled depression and anxiety before the arrival of antidepressants? The answer lies in the use of musical instruments. Music is closely linked to emotions. Music can make you feel calm, make you feel sad, happy or make you dance. Similarly, our emotional and physical state is reflected in our sound. When we are sad, our sound is different, it is different when we're happy, different when we're relaxed, etc.

Music seems to be as old as humans. In India, the dholak, tabla or drums are used during worship of gods, festivals and social events. In African countries, djembe are used to create the music for community drum circles around the fire. Almost every country on the planet uses some kind of drum or other musical instrument during community events or during celebration. Music is such an integral part of human life. A community event without music is like a movie without music. Music is the symbol of celebration, be it a harvest, a kill after a successful hunt, a wedding, a victory or whatever. All these occasions are celebrated with music. Music elevates the mood and helps us forget sadness.

A sound is basically a vibration that creates a wave of pressure that travels through air, water or solids. The best way to feel the vibrations of sound is to shut all the windows of your car and increase the volume of the stereo. You will feel the vibrations everywhere in the car. Depending on the volume, the vibrations vary. There are certain sounds that the human ear cannot hear because of its limitations.

Everything in the universe has its own rhythm and vibration. There are vibrations at the atomic level and there are vibrations among planets. There is a rhythm in the way breath and heartbeats cause vibrations, and there is the sound that Is created by vibrations. Rhythmic vibrations create balance and harmony, while disturbed rhythm creates imbalance. In an orchestra, instruments playing synchronously create music, but the same instruments, when not in sync, create noise.

Sound is a powerful healing force. Suppressed emotions and desires are stored as toxins in our mind. When we use sound consciously, we can create a profound effect on our mind. Vibrations created by sound from the throat travel through tissues all the way up to the brain, and down to the lungs and heart. These vibrations help to open up energy channels, stimulate fluids and massage tissues and cells. Many studies have shown that brainwaves are influenced by sound, music, chanting and meditation. Mantras are used extensively for healing.

Nāda yoga brings the healing effect of sound to our thoughts, emotions and body. It is all about bringing harmony and balance in various rhythms into our body with the help of vibrations of sound. Nāda yoga harnesses this property of sound. It helps relieve tension, high blood pressure, insomnia and a negative mind state, as well as evoking the deeply restorative and relaxing alpha and theta brainwave patterns.

Nāda is sound and yoga in union. Nāda yoga is creating union of the mind, body and soul using sound. It is considered as one of the most effective forms of meditation to calm the mind.

There are four levels of Nāda yoga:

1. **Vaikhari:** this is the sound we use to communicate with each other. It is the audible sound that can be heard by the human ear. It is the sound of speech, song and when two things strike each other (e.g., cymbals). This sound helps in creating one-pointed concentration to meditate. When we completely focus on the sound of a flute, harp or harmonium it helps to achieve one-pointed concentration.

2. **Madhyama:** this is mental sound and is more subtle than vaikhari. When we create the sound in our mind

before we make it, with the help of the throat, this is called madhyama. Since the sound is created by our own mind, it can only be heard by our own mind. When we recite a song in our head without making any sound it is called madhyama.

3. **Pashyanti:** this is subconscious sound or what is known as a visual sound. When we see a video of the wave without sound, we make that sound in our head through imagination based on the sound experience stored in our memory. When we dream or hear a sound without it being produced; e.g., when you hear your loved one calling you even when they're not around, it's called pashyanti. In this case you visualise the sound.

4. **Para:** this is a transcendent sound that is beyond the senses and the mind. The para voice gives birth to root ideas or germ thoughts. It is the first manifestation of voice.

Chanting or singing keeps the mind away from idle thoughts and mind chatter. Repetition of words take the shape of sound and other thoughts disappear. When we make a rhythmic sound, it regulates our breath, creates vibration in our throat and the rest of the body, which energises the body. The absence of thoughts, and the vibration of sound, bring calmness to the mind, helping it relax. Repeating the same sound constantly doesn't leave any space in the mind for any other thoughts. Parents always ask kids to read out loud. When you read out loud, the mind automatically focuses on the sound, helping you to concentrate and memorise.

Just like there are some sounds that make you feel irritated, certain sounds make you feel good and certain sounds help heal emotional wounds. Listening to a song can easily take you back in the past and associate with memories.

You can experience the vibrational property of sound by pronouncing the word "OM".

You can pronounce the letters in this word without using your tongue:

ahhh oooooo mmmmmm

That's why it is also treated as an initial sound. This is a most common sound that babies start making when they try to make sound.

The healing property of sound can easily be experienced when an ailing mother hears the voice of her child after a long time, or when we hear good news. Certain types of sound excite us and make us shake our bodies, while other types of sound help us to just relax and calm down.

Vibrations and the power of sound can be easily seen with the help of a Tibetan singing bowl. They are made of a mixture of different metals and make a calming sound. If you fill the bowl with water and rotate a wooden stick on the edges of the bowl, it makes a sound. Those sound waves pass through the water inside the bowl, making the water vibrate, which looks as though the water is being boiled and can be seen with the naked eye. Tibetan singing bowls' sound healing uses the same concept in healing the human mind. The sound is made close to your body. As the majority of the body is water, the sound makes subtle vibrations in the body, creating a healing effect.

"The sound of mantras is not mere repeating of formulas but yoga of the mouth."

Healing through nature

"Nature has the power to heal, not the physician."

The different kinds of teas, such as green tea, Darjeeling or Japanese tea, have different effects on our mood. Different fragrances also have different effects. Different colours have different effects. Trees are a combination of taste, smell and colour, which will have a combined effect.

An experiment was conducted with three people. They were all given one flower each. The first person looked at the flower and didn't react. He was still thinking about his next career move. The second person looked at the flower and appreciated the beauty of it. The third person looked at the flower and touched the petals, observed the colour combinations, colour of the pollen and the butterflies around the flower, and took a selfie.

The first person looked at the flower and his response was to still think about something else, so he didn't get anything from the experience. The second person looked at the flower and their response was appreciation. She felt the beauty of the flower. The third person's response was creative as he admired the beauty and also appreciated the colours of the petals and the texture. His creative response made him part of nature. A lot depends on your response. *You will receive what you give.*

Trees and forests are an integral part of human existence. Trees produce oxygen and absorb carbon dioxide, produce food for us, and their parts are used for various purposes. These are well-known facts. Lesser known or, rather, not acknowledged is the fact that trees are great healers. Since time immemorial, trees have been worshipped in many traditions. Now science has proven the healing properties of trees.

In 1980, Japan introduced a concept called shinrin-yoku. It literally means "forest bathing" and is about nature therapy. Shinrin-yoku acts as natural aromatherapy. The concept was introduced to avoid Karoshi; this is, death by work. Nowadays, work pressures cause stress, resulting in severe health issues. Forest bathing is actually going into a forest or park and feeling the effect of trees. Trees release compounds called phytoncides, which you inhale during the walk through the woods. Many studies have suggested that these phytoncides help to increase and stimulate the activity of white blood cells, our natural killer cells. These cells help to fight infection and are critical for a healthy immune system.

It's a simple process. Take some time out from your schedule. Even a fifteen-minute walk has a powerful effect. Leave behind your phone and other electronic gadgets. If you're going in a group, make a pact that you will not interact during the walk. Walk through the trees. Feel nature. Observe the swaying of the branches, listen to the wind passing through the branches, go close to the trees and touch their trunks, feel the textures, look at the flowers, look at the combination of colours, feel the originality of our creator, look at the pollen, look at the bees who're trying to pick the best from the heart of the flower, feel the freshness, pick up a petal or leaf, rub it in your palm, smell the fresh fragrance, see the colour that it leaves on your palm, look at the height of the trees, look at the birds flitting between its branches, and become part of the trees. Keep observing other trees and plants in the same way. At the end of the walk sit quietly, close your eyes. Feel the effect of the trees around you with closed eyes. Meditate.

This simple process has a profound effect on your body. It has been proven that this activity:

- helps to reduce blood pressure
- reduces heartrate
- reduces anxiety
- reduces stress

- increases concentration
- brings clarity of thought
- helps you feel happy.

Japan has many certified shinrin-yoku paths, and even doctors recommend going for forest bathing regularly.

Flowers have importance in almost all celebrations. The kiku flower features as an imperial seal of Japan. Representing rejuvenation and longevity, the flower is emblazoned across every Japanese passport as the symbol of the nation. The 18th century Indian poet Sant Tukaram has described trees and plants as our relatives. In a poem he mentions that when you are surrounded by trees, solitude doesn't allow any bad thoughts and habits to enter your mind. Surrounding heals your body. You get to spend time with yourself, which has tremendous benefits.

Fresh air:

The longer you stay inside your air-conditioned office, you may experience headaches, sleepiness, a low attention span and a general sense of feeling unwell. If you have a heated argument with colleagues and feel stressed, you may decide to go outside to get some fresh air. Stepping out of the office will definitely bring about a change in your mood as you step into a different environment, and that helps to create some distraction from what you want to get away from. If you go to the beach, a river, waterfall or park, then there is much more in the environment that can help to reduces stress and anxiety. There is fresh air.

So what is this fresh air? It's all about ions. Ions are charged particles in the air; some are negatively charged, and some are positively charged. Negative ions are oxygen atoms charged with an extra electron. Negative ions are beneficial for the human body. They are in plentiful supply in natural settings, and are dangerously low in the average air-conditioned office, over-heated home or stuffy car. You will find the highest concentrations of negative ions in natural, clean air.

Negative ions are produced through water molecules, which is why they are in such beautifully abundant supply near fresh, flowing water, such as rivers, streams, seas and waterfalls. This also explains how refreshing it can be to have a shower, swim or to take a bath when we are feeling exhausted. This is the atmospheric form of energy, which we assimilate through breathing, the chi in Chinese chi-gong and prana in India.

This is one reason why hermits and yogis in India traditionally preferred to live and practise in high mountains where prana is always strong, stable and pure.

Feel the calmness of moonlight.

Feel the freshness of the first rays of the sun.

Feel the melody in the chirping sound of birds.

Look around at the beauty of flowers, trees, mountains and the ocean.

Then you don't need to learn to meditate.

Flower mindfulness:

This is an easy way to practise mindfulness.

Pick up any flower. Observe the shape of the flower, look at how many petals it has: is every petal the same shape? Look at the colour combination of every petal, look at the stem and how it connects to the petals. Look at the difference in colours of the petal and stem, look at the design of the petals, look inside the flower, look at the composition inside the flower, look at the filaments, look at the anthers on top of each filament, gently touch the petals, feel their softness with your fingers, gently smell the fragrance, take a deep breath while smelling the flower. When you exhale, feel the movement of petals because of airflow from your nose. Close your eyes and deeply inhale and exhale a couple of times. Feel the air with fragrance going deep into your lungs.

"Look deep into nature, and then you will understand everything better." —Einstein

Healing through water

The human body is made up of seventy percent water.

Water is the basis for blood, gastric juices, bile, pancreatic fluid and several other fluids in the digestive system of the human body. Just as water irrigates a farm through canals, blood irrigates the body through the circulatory system. The human body is made up of cells, and every cell is made up of seventy percent water. So this means that water is the most important part of our body. In order to have healthy cells in our body, we need to have enough water.

Water is a panacea. When you are stressed, drink a glass of water; if you are feeling hot, take a cool shower, etc. Just as polluted water can cause disease, sufficient pure water in the body helps to cure many diseases. You will be surprised to know how many diseases are linked to the deficiency of water. Water helps to carry nutrients all over the body to keep all the organs healthy. It also helps to carry waste outside the body in terms of urine. Water also maintains the required body temperature through sweat. Water helps to maintain the pH level of blood. Water and ionised minerals are the two most important nutrients of the human body. Hermits prefer the Himalayan spring water as it is loaded with calcium, ionised minerals and is rich in oxygen, which minimises the need for solid food to a great extent.

Water helps to cleanse and purify the body both internally and externally. When inside the body, water directly impacts the internal organs. Similarly, water has an impact externally as well. When we immerse our body in water, we feel weightlessness as we float. The way we feel this lightness externally, the similar impact is experienced by internal organs. Most of the time we are either in a sitting, standing or sleeping position. Because of the gravitational force, organs feel the pull towards the ground. When our body is in water floating, the organs don't feel that pull from the ground. This helps organs to reposition or adjust themselves if there is any slight dislocation. It also relaxes organs as they feel less gravitational force.

"Drink a glass of water, take a dip in water and heal yourself."

Healing through aroma

Aroma holds tremendous power to create an impact on our health and mind. Just as some smells can give you a headache and nausea, some fragrances have the power to make you feel fresh and rejuvenated. When you visit a fruit shop and smell the sweet smell of mangoes, your mouth automatically salivates, stimulating your senses. It means a smell has the power to stimulate juices in your body. When you smell a flower, you automatically tend to close your eyes and try to take a deep breath, as if you want to smell as much as possible in one go. See the relaxation on your face after you smell your favourite flower. It means smell has the power to dominate senses and attract the mind. When you have a body massage, essential oils create a calming and relaxing effect on your body and mind using their aromatic healing properties.

Some of the commonly used essential oils and their benefits include the following.

Essential oil	Benefits/cure
Lavender	Insomnia, pain relief, hair care, blood circulation, indigestion, relaxation
Lemongrass	Stress relief, fights depression, reduces body odour
Lime	Boosts appetite
Orange	Uplifts mood
Patchouli	Reduces emotional and nervous disorders
Peppermint	Clears congestion and eases breathing
Rose	Helps sexual disorders
Rosemary	Mental disorders, depression, respiratory disorders
Rosewood	Promotes sexual arousal, stimulates gland discharges, cures headaches
Sandalwood	Memory booster, cough and cold relief, lowers blood pressure
Tea tree	Inhibits bacterial, viral infections
Ylang ylang	Various sexual disorders, reduces blood pressure, soothes inflammation and reduces the severity of nervous disorders
Basil	Pain relief, cures indigestion

Healing through love

"The things that are invisible to you are often the things that most surround you."

—John Hassel

A commonly known and understood concept of love is love between two people. Love is an emotion and need not always be between two people. The way you love a person, you can also love an animal and a tree as well. That's why the terms animal lover or tree lover exist. Just as humans have emotions, animals have emotions, and there are many theories that advocate that trees have emotions, too, and that they react to human emotions. Animals don't fake love.

Whether you love yourself or others fully, the truth is, love heals.

What is love? It is an emotion. Where would that be? Inside of you. If love is inside us, why do we look outside for it?

Loving is one thing, and being loved is another thing. No one can stop you from loving as that is your emotion. Being loved is another thing where we expect someone else to love us. Although opposite poles attract in magnets, this isn't the case with emotions. Love attracts love and hatred attracts hatred. If you have love in your heart, you will receive love in return. The confusion arises when we expect material things under the pretext of love, and if we don't get them we assume that the person doesn't love us. So we start hating that person and, in return, we start getting hatred and we spoil the relationship. We need to differentiate between love and material things. The expectation of material things separates people, not the expectation of love.

When we see an infant we feel love in our heart, which brings joy to ourselves. An infant may not react to you, but you would still be happy because you have love for the infant in your heart.

If the infant responds with a smile, that is the love you get from them, which makes you happier. You don't expect any other material things from the infant, so it's pure love. That's why we call mother's love the purest form of love. As we grow up, we love people around us but we attach material expectations to that love, and, if not met, we develop a hatred for them. The same is applicable in the corporate environment. We already have love inside us, we just need to open it up for people around us, and in return receive that love. Giving a smile or wishing a colleague well, even though you had a heated discussion on a previous day, is a form of love.

When we keep hatred for someone in our heart, the other person doesn't lose anything, but we lose the beautiful emotion in our heart called love. How can you love yourself and hate others?

Yale University cancer surgeon Dr Bernie Siegel, in his book *Love, Medicine and Miracles*, talks about the power of love in the healing process. Dr Siegel writes: "If I told patients to raise their blood levels of globulins or killer T cells, no one would know how. But if I can teach them to love themselves and others fully, the same changes happen automatically. The truth is: love heals."

A lack of love is one of the major causes of depression. Depression puts pressure on the immune system, causing many diseases. So a lack of love is responsible for many diseases.

All you need is love. A small step when repeated a million times makes a huge difference. Love conquers fear. Whenever there is fear in the mind, a feeling of unconditional love will diminish that fear. Meditation will melt anger. The absence of anger automatically fills the heart with love. A heart full of love brings happiness, and happiness brings health. Anger is like a solid ice cube. It makes us stiff and when angry we can't think of anything else. When we meditate, it's like this ice cube melts away into the water and eventually becomes vapours and disappears.

The mind is relaxed in the absence of anger.

Healing through Knowledge

Knowledge is one of the most important healing aids. One of the three Ps of consciousness as mentioned earlier in this book, is perceive. It is about what we perceive. It is not necessary that every time we pick the right knowledge. It's like believing in rumours. When we believe a rumour, it may not be true but we still pick that knowledge and believe in it. Getting the right knowledge is important and can help you to understand the reality. In an office environment, we keep assuming many things without always understanding the facts, which creates stress and anxiety. It's always good to get the facts before we respond to a situation. Knowledge Management plays an important role in success of an organisation. Imagine launching a new product without doing a market study. There will be a high chance of failure.

If you are depressed, anxious, seek knowledge from right sources. Knowledge heals.

Healing through Food

> *"The majority of diseases can be traced back to troubles in the stomach and intestine."*

A simple fact but largely ignored is that our stomach is responsible for digesting what we eat. That is the first organ impacted by food that is difficult to digest. The large intestine is a great sewer of the body. It carries all waste material to the anus to be expelled out of the body. When this sewer is clogged, we call it constipation. An unhealthy diet is one of the major causes of constipation. This great sewer has tiny absorbent channels. When they become clogged, some of the poisonous waste material is absorbed back into the system, which leads to disease.

Your mind and body are two different things. We consume mind-altering drugs that alter the mind, but what about the body? We do this at the cost of the body. What we forget is that the same body that consumes mind-altering drugs to alter the mind, affects the mind when any part of the body is damaged. Poison in our body affects the quality of our thoughts. When you consume alcohol, you feel an impact on your mind, but consumption of excessive alcohol has a damaging effect on various parts of the body as well, such as the liver. A damaged liver will also make your mind unstable and create stress and anxiety. So we get into a vicious cycle. We use our nostrils to inhale drugs, while the nostrils are actually there to assist inhaling fresh air. We use our mouths to consume drugs and alcohol, while the mouth is to assist us to provide nutrition to our body. If an organ is misused, then the bad effects are obvious.

Not everyone consumes drugs, alcohol or other mind-altering substances. But the fact is that what we consume has an effect on the body. The things we eat and drink without awareness of their impact on the body may not be as extreme as drugs and alcohol, but they will certainly have an effect on the body as well as on the mind. What we eat affects our mental state. We've all experienced how even the thought of a disgusting thing affects our appetite. Emotions like sadness, anger and hatred also equally impact the appetite. Emotional imbalance causes improper digestion. This results in less nourishment for our body. Less nourishment can have a cascading effect throughout the body. We ignore these facts and boast about working lunches in the office. Time to think about whether we really should have working lunches at the cost of our health.

"It doesn't matter how much you eat; what matters is how much you digest."

Research has proven that our body cells have a biological clock, which tells us when to sleep and when to wake up. Similarly, they also tell us when it is time for breakfast, lunch and dinner. Irregular food intake has visible side effects on the body.

The old saying goes:
> *Eat breakfast like a king,*
> *eat lunch like a rich person*
> *and eat dinner like a beggar.*

Our body needs energy throughout the day so it's important to have a nutritious breakfast that will give the body the energy it needs. A good lunch will make sure that you maintain that energy during the rest of the day. A light dinner is with the intention that the body is soon going to rest throughout the night, and this helps to regulate the metabolic mechanism. So it's a perfect cycle of twelve hours of eating during the day and twelve hours of abstaining from food during the night.

Often, we break the cycle and do not listen to the requirements of the body. Eating late at night has a severe impact on the body and sleep. Doctors always advise you to maintain the timing of food intake. We often skip lunches during office hours or have late lunches, stressing the body and mind. Although food has healing properties, food can act as a poison as well. That's where the food poisoning term originates. We get food poisoning because of eating the wrong food. White sugar is termed a poison as the excess consumption of it leads to many fatal diseases. There are many eating habits we follow just because we like the food. It may harm our body but we still consume it.

When we are ill, doctors advise us to eat certain types of food and avoid certain types of food. This itself is the biggest testimony that food heals.

Healing through food is very simple:

- Follow a twelve-hour cycle: twelve hours of the day with regular time to eat; twelve hours at night to abstain from eating.
- Be mindful of what you consume; vegetables and fruits will always be winners.

When we eat food, question whether what we eat is for the body or for the senses. There is a huge difference in what's needed for the body and what our senses like. That's where the problem lies. Whatever we eat, our body should say thank you, not the senses.

"We are what we eat."

As per yogic practices, nature—a primary force of life—is composed of three qualities or principles: sattva (tranquil or subtle energy), rajas (active energy) and tamas (inertia or dullness).

- Sattvic food is fresh, properly cooked.
- Rajasic food is salty, spicy, fried.
- Tamasic food is stale, over-processed.

What we eat also decides what kind of sleep we get. Sattvic food causes sattvic sleep (sleep that brings lightness, brightness and freshness); rajasic food causes rajasic sleep (disturbed, irritated, restless); and tamasic food causes tamasic sleep (feeling heavy, lethargic and dull after sleep).

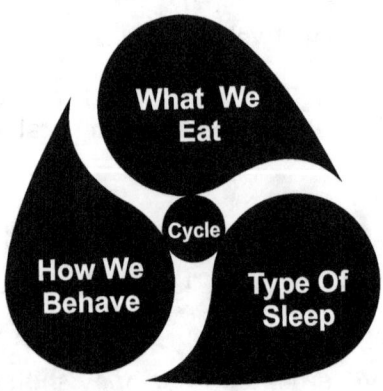

Fig.- Cycle of sleep, Behaviour & food

We return to innocence in sleep. Sattvic food helps to transform this innocence into a positive state of mind while awake. The goal of yogic practices is to have sattvic sleep. So it is important to choose what we eat. Yogic practices do not let tamasic nature dominate sattvic.

The human body uses enzymes in almost all metabolic and biological activities. Sattvic food provides enzymes for the body. The body creates enzymes using protein, minerals and energy. When the body receives enzymes through food, there is less need to produce enzymes within the body. Unfortunately, the food we eat is often acidic, over-processed and lacks the

244

enzymes needed by the body. In such cases, the body has to work extra hard to create the required enzymes. Acidic food also disturbs the pH level of the blood. This needs to be maintained to help blood carry energy effectively. Acidic food causes the stagnation of energy. It also causes chronic acidosis of the blood and intercellular food, which is the main contributing factor to many degenerative diseases, such as high blood pressure, immune deficiency and cancer.

One more way to regulate diet and balance the entire digestive system is abstinence of food at regular intervals. This gives the digestive system time to slow down and recover from the losses.

Healing through art

Art is another form of meditation. When you are involved in art, you awaken the creative side of you, which dominates all other aspects. Creativity fills your mind, replacing all other emotions. It could be any form of art that appeals to your mind: painting, writing, singing, dancing, etc. Art brings enjoyment, fun and playfulness. These things have the potential to tame fear and worry, which are negative contributors to any health challenge you're faced with.

The mind is like a small passage. At any given point in time, only a limited number of thoughts can pass through it. If there are existing thoughts in the mind, new thoughts cannot enter unless you make space for them. When you are stressed and practise art, it means you are asking thoughts that are causing stress to

245

step aside and make way for creative thoughts. When creative thoughts occupy the mind, this reduces the effect of stress and helps in the healing process.

You don't need to be an artist to heal through art, you just need to try the art and things will follow automatically. The satisfaction of creating something on your own has its own joy as you become the creator.

Art therapy also works well even if you feel that you're not stressed. In our day-to-day mundane life, we get used to routine activities and we become less responsive to things around us. When we learn a new thing, our mind gets active with increased concentration. The curiosity of learning a new thing and a sense of accomplishment after doing new things helps to release the feel-good hormones, which help us to stay positive and reduce negative emotions.

Art reveals emotions trapped inside the mind. Have you noticed how your handwriting changes with emotions? You can make out subtle changes in your handwriting based on your emotions at the time of writing, such as sadness, joy and anger. Art brings out emotions. If you give a crayon to a toddler, they draw what's in their mind. But when you give the same crayon to an adult, what he draws will be completely different. It's not the skill that matters, it's what is in your mind that matters.

When you write a story, paint a picture or dance, all these activities will reflect your mood. So when you practise art, it will give you a way to express the emotions stuck in your mind, thus relaxing the mind. Art increases concentration, and increased concentration helps to stabilise a chaotic mind.

When my friend Sophie lost her job, terrible insomnia and headaches started daunting her. She had two young kids to look after. A friend suggested she buy some watercolour paints to avoid boredom and stress. One night, at around 3 am when she couldn't stop tossing in bed because of stress, she took out her paints, picked up a pebble from her backyard, jumped online to get some ideas and began to paint the pebble. She had never done that before, but whatever she was painting made her feel better. Her mind became more creative and she no longer needed online inspiration. She started coming up with her own ideas of rock painting. She now sells her rock paintings online, which has been an important part of her recovery. Sophie found art therapy so beneficial in her recovery that the art has become an integral part of her life now. Art has given Sophie back her power to live a stress-free life.

People suffering from mental health often feel isolated because no one else understands what is going on inside of them. For them, art becomes a connection to express their feelings to the external world, which is an important part of healing.

There is a lot of evidence showing the effectiveness of art therapy. A 2017 study from Sweden's University of Gothenburg found that after a ten-hour-long art therapy session, patients suffering from moderate to severe depression improved on an average of almost five steps on a rating scale used for depression. Research published in 2016 in the *Journal of the American Art Therapy Association* found that forty-five minutes of art-making reduces levels of the stress hormone cortisol; therefore, increasing the body's relaxation response. Evidence reported in *The Arts in Psychotherapy* journal confirmed that engaging in art for as little as three minutes activates the brain's reward pathways. "Positive emotions play a tremendous role in relieving many symptoms," says Noah Hass-Cohen, author of *Art Therapy and the Neuroscience of Relationships, Creativity, and Resiliency: Skills and Practices*. There is also evidence that art therapy helps patients with dementia and significantly alleviates symptoms of psychological trauma.

"Your wound is probably not your fault, but your healing is your responsibility."

—Denice Frohman

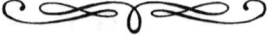

When you become a corporate yogi, you don't give up anything. You just stop taking what is not needed by your body, such as stress and anxiety.

We all know that our health is important. What we ignore is the strong relationship between physical health and the mind. Yogic practices help us to understand this relationship between physical health and the mind, and bring joy into our life.

When a cruise ship needs to turn, it does so by slowly changing course. Yoga does the same thing with our life and mind. Just like we may not notice the turning of the cruise ship, eventually it turns by making small movements. Yogic practices create small differences at a time, eventually creating a huge difference. Yoga creates a positive impact on our body and mind.

.

About the author

Ravindra Puri is an Indian-Australian, business excellence professional and yoga practitioner based in Sydney. His corporate life is associated with large organisations in India and Australia. He was first exposed to yogic practices in a "Happiness Program" run by the Art of Living foundation, established by yoga guru Sri Sri Ravi Shankar.

Just like most people in the world, Ravindra has had his share of troubles in life. Yogic practices have helped him to sail through the turbulent times, and through this "The Book of a Corporate Yogi" was born.

Author can be reached at-

2018rdp@gmail.com

"The book of a corporate yogi"

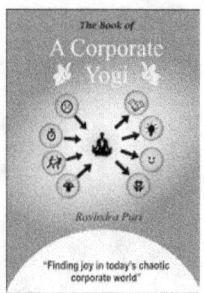

A perfect gift

For

Someone you care

For bulk/Corporate orders, please write to-

2018rdp@gmail.com